community mental health:

target populations

ANN WOLBERT BURGESS, R.N., D.N.Sc.
*Associate Professor and Coordinator
Graduate Program in Community Health Nursing
Boston College, Chestnut Hill
Massachusetts*

AARON LAZARE, M.D.
*Associate Professor of Psychiatry
at the Massachusetts General Hospital,
Harvard Medical School
Director of Outpatient Psychiatry
Massachusetts General Hospital*

PRENTICE-HALL, INC., Englewood Cliffs, New Jersey

Library of Congress Cataloging in Publication Data

Burgess, Ann Wolbert.
   Community mental health.

   Includes bibliographical references and index.
   1. Community mental health services. 2. Crisis
intervention (Psychiatry) 3. Personality, Disorders of.
4. Psychic trauma. I. Lazare, Aaron, joint author.
II. Title. [DNLM: 1. Community mental health
services. WM30 B955c]
RA790.B787   362.2'04'25   75-43886
ISBN 0-13-153148-4

We dedicate this book
to our fathers,
John N. Wolbert and H. Benjamin Lazare

10 9 8 7 6 5 4 3 2 1

Printed in the United States of America

PRENTICE-HALL INTERNATIONAL, INC., *London*
PRENTICE-HALL OF AUSTRALIA PTY. LIMITED, *Sydney*
PRENTICE-HALL OF CANADA, LTD., *Toronto*
PRENTICE-HALL OF INDIA PRIVATE LIMITED, *New Delhi*
PRENTICE-HALL OF JAPAN, INC., *Tokyo*
PRENTICE-HALL OF SOUTHEAST ASIA PTE. LTD., *Singapore*

contents

iii

foreword

In this day of multiple human problems and the growing awareness of the interrelationship of human social systems, mental
health workers, researchers, and committed citizens have pushed
away the walls of mental health institutions. "Wall-less," confused
people in distress and workers stand confronted with the swirling
complexities of the community. It is the raw awareness of the impact of this phenomenon that distinguishes Drs. Burgess and
Lazare's text from other books on community mental health. The
first five chapters underscore their approach to community mental
health. They present with great success an integrated clinical approach, backed by relevant paradigms of mental health, illness,
social process, and human development proposed by other
clinicians, theoreticians, and researchers. Their text is strengthened
by their contributors. In addition, they demonstrate the usefulness of their clinical approaches in the sections dealing with sex
and violence. True to their word, they are willing to share how
they formulated their clinical hypotheses, initiated their interventions, and evaluated outcomes.

In conclusion, I find their text extremely important for beginning community practitioners because it does deal with the clinical issues in a head-on manner.

Oh, how protective those state mental hospital walls have been to staff! It is just another matter when you go into a home and talk with a troubled teenager who has been expelled from school and is addicted to drugs, or to a mother with six young children who is having difficulty coping with an abusive and alcoholic husband, or to a child victim of sexual assault.

Burgess and Lazare know what is encountered within the community, and they assist the practitioner in understanding how multiple theories of intervention in human behavioral disorders make sense in clinical community practice.

Carol R. Hartman, R.N., D.N. Sc.
Associate Professor and Coordinator
Graduate Program in Psychiatric Nursing
Boston College

preface

The demands for mental health services, fostered by the community health movement, require that professionals pay attention to and care for populations that have been previously neglected and/or difficult to treat. In an attempt to approach this problem we have set out to write a textbook with two major foci: (1) a conceptual approach to the problem, and (2) the target populations themselves.

In Part One, "Conceptual Framework," we describe how clinicians can use biologic, psychologic, social, and behavioral approaches to human behavior in order to understand all dimensions of the clinical problem most fully. The interview for community settings is based on this approach. We then redefine the relationship between the helper and client in mental health situations. The client is treated as a customer of mental health services—a customer whose rights should be taken quite seriously because the request for care is usually reasonable and always negotiable. This "customer relationship" makes the client more understandable and diminishes the clinician's sense of helplessness.

Concepts and patterns of crises are discussed, because very often the client comes to a mental health facility in a crisis state. To complete Part One, issues in mental health consultation are presented to assist clinicians who are called upon to discuss and interpret the mental health issues to members of the community.

In Part Two, "Target Populations," we have used the above conceptual framework to study and understand groups of people who have been previously neglected both in clinical practice and in the professional literature. We believe that the humanistic traditions of our mental health professions commit us to care for the bereaved, the infertile, the alcoholic, the drug abusers, the suicidal, the sexual offenders, the victims of violence and sexual trauma, and the prostitute. Within the chapters that deal with those target populations we attempt to apply the conceptual framework to present a new model of care for these groups. We hope that this framework will be used for teaching clinicians to study other neglected target populations in order to increase clinical skills in aiding people in mental health distress.

We sought experts to present certain of the target population groups. Chapter 7, "The Infertile Couple," was written by Barbara Eck Menning, who is Director of *Resolve*, a Boston-based self-help organization for infertile people. She is also a nurse-educator and has taught as a maternal-child health nursing instructor in Afghanistan and at Northeastern University in Boston.

Chapter 8, "Alcoholism in the Community," and Chapter 9, "The Drug Abuser," were written by John A. Renner, Jr., who is Director of the Alcohol Clinic and Drug Treatment Program at Massachusetts General Hospital. He is an Instructor in Psychiatry at Harvard Medical School and brings administrative, clinical, and theoretical expertise to these issues.

Chapter 12, "Aggressive Sexual Offenders: Diagnosis and Treatment," was written by A. Nicholas Groth and Murray L. Cohen. Dr. Groth is Chief Psychologist, Massachusetts Department of Mental Health, Division of Legal Medicine and is on the faculty of both Simmons College and Northeastern University in Boston. Dr. Cohen is Professor and Chairman of the Clinical-Community Psychology Program at Boston University and has been consultant to the Massachusetts Treatment Center since its inception. Drs. Groth and Cohen have been involved for many years in evaluation, treatment, and clinical research of sexually violent men. The themes of their contributions derive from those clinical activities and reflect the very particular stance of the clinician in his relationships with the patient-offender and with various social institutions.

We have written this book for the interdisciplinary groups of health care providers—nurses, physicians, psychologists, social workers, educators, clergy—who often see the clients of the target populations. Mental health professionals will be constantly faced with the task of helping clients deal with a wide variety of trauma, losses, and crises. Applying the framework of the customer approach and the clinical negotiation to previously neglected target populations in the community is a step toward more effective treatment interventions.

We extend our appreciation to the many people with whom we have worked in the various phases of our research and practice. We especially wish to acknowledge our colleagues—Sherman Eisenthal, Lynda Lytle Holmstrom, Owen S. Surman and Linda Wasserman—who collaborated with us on the research and publications that are included in this text.

We thank Margaret Smith Hamilton, Linda Kehrli Lynett, and Carolyn J. Thomas for clinical cases cited in the book and Janet E. Cannon for typing parts of the manuscript.

We very much appreciate the manuscript review program provided by our editor, Harry A. McQuillen, and his assistant, Barbara Nissen-Bartlett, of Prentice-Hall, Inc. The thorough editorial production of the book was directed by Margaret G. McNeily of Prentice-Hall, Inc., who was most helpful in the final details of the project.

Our warmest thanks go to our children, Elizabeth, Benton, Clayton, and Sarah Burgess; Jacqueline, Samuel, Sarah, Thomas, Hien, Robert, and David Lazare. And we are deeply appreciative of the discussions, suggestions, and support of Allen G. Burgess and Louise C. Lazare throughout the project.

Ann Wolbert Burgess
Aaron Lazare

Boston, Massachusetts

I
conceptual framework

A multidimensional model for mental health practice is described and presented throughout this book. A major concept, the customer approach to patienthood, shows how the health seeker can relate to the provider. This concept, which ensures that the rights of health seekers are taken seriously, treats patients as customers of mental health services by recognizing that patients' requests for care are usually reasonable and always negotiable. An interview for community settings describes a method for systematic check ing that covers all areas of possible concern in the interview. Crisis diagnosis and mental health consultation are important concepts in an overall framework for practice.

1

a multidimensional approach
to psychopathology

Many people find it difficult to understand how a psychiatric clinician selects relevant clinical data, formulates a case, and chooses a treatment program. In the psychiatrically ill patient, is it the symptom complex, the "unconscious conflict," or the abnormality in family interactions that contains the key to clinical decision making? How is it that one clinician will emphasize electroconvulsive therapy or tricyclic antidepressants, another, individual therapy, and a third, family therapy—all for apparently similar patients? Why is it apparently easier to formulate and implement a treatment plan for a patient suffering from a medical illness such as congestive heart failure?

One major reason for the difficulty in understanding psychiatric thinking is that several different conceptual models are implicitly used in the clinical formulation but rarely identified as

This chapter is adapted from Aaron Lazare, "Hidden Conceptual Models in Clinical Psychiatry," *New England Journal of Medicine* 288, No. 7 (February 15, 1973), 345–351. Copyright 1973 by the New England Journal of Medicine, and used with permission.

such. The four most common models are the biologic, the psychologic, the behavioral, and the social. When a patient is treated, the kind of history obtained, the meaning assigned to certain historical facts, and the treatment modalities most often chosen depend on what model or combination of models is employed. These points are illustrated by four case histories of the same middle-aged depressed female patient. Each history is formulated in terms of one of the four conceptual models.

Case History — Biologic Model

Mrs. J., a 53-year-old widow, gave a history of a depressive syndrome. During the past few months she had lost 20 lb in weight, had early morning awakening, and had a diurnal variation in mood manifested by feeling better as the day went on. She described herself as feeling hopeless, helpless, and worthless. There was some retardation of speech. She denied suicidal intent and presented no evidence of delusions or paranoid ideation. Twenty-three years previously a similar episode of depression had remitted spontaneously. The patient had a sister who was hospitalized for a depressive illness that responded positively to electroconvulsive treatments.

Case History — Psychologic Model

Mrs. J., a 53-year-old widow, had been depressed for a few months after the death of her husband. Although the marriage seemed happy at times, there were many stormy periods in their relation. There had been no visible signs of grief since his death. Since the funeral, she had been depressed and had lost interest in her surroundings. For no apparent reason she blamed herself for minor events of the past. Sometimes she criticized herself for traits that characterized her husband more than herself. She had had a similar reaction after the death of her mother 23 years previously, when she and her mother had lived together. From the family history, it could be inferred that the relation was characterized by hostile dependency. Six months after her mother's death, the patient married. She seemed intelligent and motivated for treatment, and had considered psychotherapy in the past to gain a better understanding of herself.

Case History — Behavioral Model

Mrs. J., a 53-year-old widow gave a history of depressive behaviors of anorexia, insomnia, feelings of hopelessness, helplessness, and worthlessness. These behaviors had begun shortly after the death of her husband. Throughout the marriage, he had been a continuous source of reinforcement to the patient. This quality of the husband's interaction with his wife had been evident since the marriage, at a time when the patient was still depressed after her mother's death. The family stated that the husband had always ignored the patient's demands and pleas of helplessness while responding actively to the more positive aspects of her personality. After his death, she began to complain to her children about her loss of appetite and her sense of helplessness. They responded to these complaints with frequent visits and telephone calls, but the depressive behavior only worsened.

Case History — Social Model

Mrs. J., a 53-year-old widow, had been depressed during the past few months since the death of her husband. He had been the major figure in her life, and his loss has left her feeling lonely and isolated. After his death, she moved to a small apartment, which was some distance from her old neighborhood. Although she was satisfied with her new quarters, she found the community strange. Furthermore, she did not have access to public transportation, which would have enabled her to visit her old friends, children, and grandchildren. Since her husband's death, old strains between the patient and her children had been aggravated.

These four histories could each have been elicited from the same patient by four different clinicians, each employing a different conceptual model in formulating the case. This use by clinicians of different conceptual models often bewilders the student, who sees patients with similar symptoms diagnosed and treated differently. Clinicians themselves, by using one model to the exclusion of others, unnecessarily limit new treatment options.

This chapter will first describe the four most frequently employed conceptual models for the diagnosis of psychiatric illness by reference to the histories cited above. It will then attempt to show how in everyday practice the decision to use one or a combination of models is implicitly determined by the interplay of physician, patient, and clinical situation. By making explicit the implicit, the decision-making process in clinical psychiatry can become more rational, a broader range of treatment modalities should be made available, and the communication between clinicians should be enhanced.

FOUR MAJOR MODELS

The Biologic Model

The biologic (or medical) model views psychiatric illnesses as diseases like any others. For each disease, it is supposed that there eventually will be found a specific cause related to the functional anatomy of the brain.[1] * The clinician using the biologic model is primarily concerned with etiology, pathogenesis, signs and symptoms, differential diagnosis, treatment, and prognosis. Knowing the syndrome or disease determines the treatment. While addressing patients with proper medical respect, the clinician keeps a distance so as to maintain objectivity.

Consider the case history according to the biologic model. The clinician, in eliciting the history of the symptom picture, observes a group of symptoms consistent with the cluster of endogenous depression.[2,3] The current syndrome, the earlier episode of depression, and the family history make the diagnosis of manic-depressive illness (depressed type) the most probable. The patient's relation with her family, her ambivalence toward her husband, and her motivation to understand her illness are interesting, and perhaps even relevant, but not central to the recognition of the illness. Antidepressant medications or electroconvulsive treatments will be the treatment of choice. The patient will be told that she is suffering from a depression, a psychiatric illness, which is not uncommon in her age group. The illness is time limited and, with proper treatment, has a favorable prognosis.

The Psychologic Model

According to the psychologic model, the developmental impasse, the early deprivation, the distortions in early relations, and the confused communication between parent and child lead to the adult neuroses and vulnerabilities to certain stresses. As a result of these psychologic determinants, we see patients who distort reality, who are prone to depression, who avoid heterosexuality, or who fear success. The social setting may be changed, psychotropic drugs may be given, but the abnormality remains because the personality is abnormal.

Therapy consists of clarifying the psychologic meaning of events, feelings, and behaviors. The patient is taught how to experience appropriate feelings and how to bear "unbearable" feelings.[4] Forgotten events may be remembered, reexperienced, and then put into perspective so that the patient can be freed to see current situations as they really are. As a result, growth and maturity are enhanced.

Most important to the therapeutic situation is the clinician-

---

*Superscript numbers in this chapter refer to numbered references at end of this chapter.

patient relation. It is the therapeutic alliance between the two that will enable the patient to remember what she has not wanted to remember and to abandon familiar but pathologic ways of coping. It is through the vehicle of the therapeutic relation—by experiencing these feelings toward the therapist—that the patient will recreate some of his previous pathologic relations to important others and have the opportunity for a "corrective emotional experience."[5]

Returning to the case history—the clinician, using the psychologic model, first takes note of the problems in the marital relation. He pays special attention to the absence of grief,[6] which has psychologic meaning and is related to the patient's ambivalent feelings toward her husband. A similar reaction after her mother's death suggests the possibility of a psychologic connection between her feelings toward her husband and mother. This is reinforced by the history that she married only six months after the death of her mother. The patient's criticism of herself in terms that she had used to criticize her husband suggests Freud's concept of introjection of the lost object.[7] Since the primary modality of treatment is psychotherapy, it is a favorable sign that she is motivated to gain a better understanding of herself.

The Behavioral Model

According to the behavioral model, both neurosis and psychosis are examples of abnormal behavior that has been learned as a result of aversive events and are maintained either because they lead to positive effects or because they avoid deleterious ones. The overt symptoms are the ones that require treatment since they themselves are the problem and not secondary manifestations of disease or unconscious conflict. The typical therapeutic course includes: (1) determining the behavior to be modified; (2) establishing the conditions under which the behavior occurs; (3) determining the factors responsible for the persistence of the behavior; (4) selecting a set of treatment conditions; and (5) arranging a schedule of retraining. The conditions that precede the behavior may be modified by such technics as desensitization, reciprocal inhibition, and conditioned avoidance. The conditions that result from the behavior may be modified by positive reinforcement, negative reinforcement, aversive conditioning, and extinction.[8]

Considering the case history according to the behavioral model, the clinician first identifies the pathologic behaviors of anorexia, insomnia, and feelings of helplessness. He then determines the empirical relation between the depressive behaviors and the antecedent and consequent environmental events that precipitate and maintain the depression.[9] The death of the husband, considering the history of the marriage, is interpreted as a sudden withholding of positive reinforcement of adaptive behavior. The attention received from family members inadvertently reinforces the depressive behaviors.

Treatment consists of reinforcing adaptive behaviors incompatible with depression and extinguishing depressive behaviors. The clinician may accomplish these therapeutic goals by teaching the family to respond positively to the adaptive behavior instead of the depressive behavior [10] or by purposefully encouraging the patient to express feelings incompatible with depression.[11]

The Social Model

The social view of psychiatric illness focuses on the way in which the individual functions in the social system. Symptoms are traced not to conflicts within the mind, not to manifestations of psychiatric disease, but to the "relationship of the individual to his manner of functioning in social situations—i.e., in the type and quality of his 'connectedness' to the groups which make up his life space."[12] Symptoms may therefore be regarded as an index of social disorder.[13-15] Accordingly, when a socially disruptive event occurs such as daughter's leaving the home, a wife's death, a geographic displacement by urban renewal, a war, or an economic depression, the resultant symptoms are seen as stemming from the social disorder.

Treatment consists of reorganizing the patient's relation to the social system or reorganizing the social system. If others do not seem to care, how can she get them to care? If the patient's behavior is irrational, how can she learn to stop acting irrationally, or how can her family better tolerate the behavior? If the therapist wants to restructure the "nuclear" social system, he may see the patient with her family. If the therapist wants to affect the broader social system, he may attempt to influence major social issues such as housing or education.

The clinician, using the social model to study the case, notices that the patient's social matrix has been altered in two ways. In the first place, she has permanently lost the one person to whom she has been closest. Secondly, by moving, she has placed herself in a situation where she has lost access to those with whom she had previously related. In individual or group therapy one could temporarily substitute a transitional social system. Simultaneously, the therapist would attempt to reestablish a social field in which she could be comfortable after discharge. To this end, he might encourage her to move to a home where she could have better access to family and old friends. He might work with the family to repair any estrangement. He might suggest a return to work. Continued individual or group therapy might help her acquire social skills that she might never have developed in the marital situation.

DETERMINATION OF THE CONCEPTUAL MODEL IN CLINICAL PRACTICE

The clinician implicitly uses one or a combination of conceptual models in evaluating and treating the patient by the process referred to as clinical judgment. He may make the selection according to the results of outcome studies. He may select the conceptual model on practical grounds: "This is the only available treatment; let's make the best of it." Sometimes he decides on ideologic grounds. In this section, we will attempt to describe some of the variables that determine the choice of conceptual model in clinical practice.

Ideology of the Therapist

Studies of the attitudes of psychotherapists toward the understanding of mental illness have concluded that several ideologies exist. Ideology here refers to a coherent system of ideas subscribed to by a subgroup of the profession as a whole. Armor and Klerman point out that ideologic factions are most likely to occur when the codified knowledge base is markedly incomplete or ambiguous about the means to be used to attain a professional goal.[16] This is precisely the position of psychiatry today.

Studies of psychiatric ideologies describe three basic orientations: biologic (somatotherapeutic, directive-organic); psychologic (psychotherapeutic, analytic-psychologic); and social (sociotherapeutic).[16-20] These studies do not explore the behavioral orientation, which, in contrast to the other three, has received its greatest impetus from psychologists. Of the ideologies described above, it must be remembered that only a small number of psychotherapists can be rigidly classified into a single ideology. More commonly, the clinician is committed in various degrees to one or more ideologies.

Diagnosis and the Effectiveness of
Somatic Treatment

Other things being equal, particular psychiatric syndromes are more apt to be viewed by one model in preference to another. The schizophrenic and manic-depressive psychoses are apt to be conceptualized primarily as biologic illness. This is supported by the mounting evidence of genetic transmission of the schizophrenias[21] and some of the depressive illnesses[22] and by the clear-cut efficacy of phenothiazines for the treatment of schizophrenia, lithium for the treatment of manic-depressive illness, and the tricyclics, monoamine oxidase inhibitors, and electroconvulsive therapy for the treatment of the endogenous depressions. In current practice, social treatments, especially in inpatient settings, are combined with the biologic approaches described above. The zeal for psychotherapeutic intervention in these syndromes has certainly lessened over the past decade, although that approach continues to enjoy considerable support.

The neuroses are more apt to be treated by the psychotherapeutic approach, although some clinicians maintain a biologic model of neurotic behavior.[23] For these disorders, syndromes are less clearly separable, there is no definite evidence of genetic transmission, and medication has less specific effects. Furthermore, the efficacy of psychotherapy in these disorders is gaining support from clinical research.[24, 25]

Clinical phenomena currently thought by many psychiatrists to be more a social disorder than a psychologic or biologic illness are drug abuse and many forms of violence. From the social perspective, changes in society, rather than massive psychotherapy programs or breakthroughs in psychopharmacology, will be necessary to effect change in these problems.

Social Class and Other Attributes of
the Patient

A number of studies have demonstrated the importance of the patient's social class in the application of psychotherapy.[26-29] Patients of the middle and upper social classes are more apt to be accepted for, and to continue in, psychotherapy. Patients of the lower and lower-middle class, in contrast, have a poorer chance of being accepted for therapy and drop out of treatment at higher rates.[30] Other patient characteristics that determine the use of psychotherapy include responsibility, verbal intelligence, psychologic mindedness, the capacity for forming a close personal relation, young adult age, history of effective adaptation before the current difficulty, likeability, and attractiveness.[31] In addition, patients treated by psychotherapy are apt to continue in treatment when their expectations are congruent with those of the therapist.[32]

Such a patient population, presenting as they often do as relatively healthy people who want help in achieving personal fulfillment (greater psychologic strength, more satisfactory relationships, comfort with their sexual identity, etc.), may be rejected by the medical psychiatrist as "not mentally ill."

Although a psychotherapeutically-oriented clinician may attempt to explain and understand most or all of pathologic and normal behavior by psychoanalytic theory, he is likely not to take patients into treatment if they want medication or advice, if they have had previous psychiatric hospitalization, if they are authoritarian in personality, if they are vulnerable to psychosis, if they are psychotic, older, or if they present a multitude of somatic complaints.[31]

Available Services

The available treatment resources are an important determinant of the choice of model. Psychotherapy clinics, especially when not overcrowded, attempt to apply psychotherapy in understanding of patients. Walk-in and emergency clinics, in responding to large numbers of patients, approach the patient from social and biologic perspectives that usually require less time from the clinician but are effective for many clinical conditions.

There are many psychiatric hospitals that specialize in the application of electroconvulsive treatments. These facilities, in their application of the biologic model, frequently overdiagnose syndromes as responsive to this form of therapy. In similar fashion, psychiatric hospitals that specialize in social (family therapy, therapeutic communities) or psychologic technics (intensive individual psychotherapy) may regard biologic treatments such as electroconvulsive treatments and psychotropic drugs as offering "only" symptomatic relief even when it is likely that such a treatment will produce marked clinical remission.

Immediacy of the Social Situation

Where the social cause is obvious, pressing, and immediate, first consideration is usually given to a social treatment. If a child is apathetic and withdrawn as a result of a continuous psychologic and physical assault at the hands of his parents, the child must initially be treated by a change in his social situation. Either the parents must change their behavior, or they must be separated from the child. If a soldier becomes psychotic in combat, the initial treatment must be his removal from the front line. Psychologic attempts at treatment during a social crisis are usually unsatisfactory.

DISCUSSION

The various conceptual models in clinical psychiatry may lead some to draw a comparison to the Tower of Babel, where confusion reigned because many languages were spoken. To the contrary, I believe the current positions of the biologic, psychologic, behavioral, and social models attest to the vitality of psychiatry as it attempts to understand the complex problems of abnormal behavior.

The biologic model, after giving psychiatry its classification of mental illness in the late nineteenth century, has provided the conceptual foundations for (1) the development and use of the antipsychotic and antidepressant medications, (2) studies of the genetic transmission of mental illness, and (3) metabolic studies of psychiatric illness, especially the depressions.[33, 34] The most important events in all the above three areas have occurred since 1950.

The psychologic model has exerted considerable influence not only on American psychiatry but also on everyday thinking. Its derivative, psychotherapy, has become a commonly accepted treatment of choice, especially for the neuroses and personality disorders. Advocates of the psychologic model, especially since World War II, have been able to translate the clinical insights derived from classical psychoanalysis and more recent developments of ego psychology into concepts that residents in nearly all training centers in the United States can use in the understanding of most psychiatric patients.

The behavioral model, resting on theoretical foundations from the early twentieth century, began its period of rapid growth in the late 1950s. Its derivative, behavior therapy, has enjoyed considerable interest in the clinical field during the relatively brief period of its existence. Behavior therapists are hopeful of offering several possible advantages to other forms of treatment, including shorter duration of treatment and applicability to a broad range of patients.

The social model, like the biologic, psychologic, and behavioral, was reawakened in the 1950s. Since that time the psychiatric ward has been viewed as a social system,[35, 36] the relation between social class and mental illness has been established, and federal legislation to provide psychiatric care for catchment areas in the community has been enacted.[37] During these years, various treatment modalities have succeeded as treatment for the mentally ill patient with minimal separation from his social milieu.

It is unfortunate that the conceptual models have remained so separate from each other. To the degree that this occurs, communications between professionals are impaired, progress requiring a broad focus is slowed, and treatment options are unnecessarily limited. There are several forces, however, that are forging the various models into a multidimensional framework.

1. Mounting evidence for the effectiveness of particular treatment does in time overwhelm partisan advocacy of a theoretical position. For example, the success of lithium in the prevention of recurrences of manic-depressive illness has led to its more widespread use in preference to wholly psychodynamic approaches.
2. Over the last two decades, the almost monolithic influence exercised by psychoanalysis on American psychiatry has waned as evidenced by appointments of chairmen of academic departments of psychiatry with more eclectic interests and a greater competence in basic research.
3. Psychiatric residents, moved by the concern for the large number of patients excluded from psychiatric consideration by the limited use of models, have insisted on broader grounding in a wide variety of treatment approaches.
4. Theoretical bridges between models point the direction toward a unified theory of human behavior. For example, attempts have been made to demonstrate how behavioral technics are involved in dynamic psychotherapy,[38, 39] how the psychoanalytic approach to symptom formation can be understood as a social process,[14] and how medical problems related to the autonomic nervous system can be approached by means of behavioral technics.[40]

Conceptual Problems

Despite these favorable trends, serious conceptual difficulties remain. Whereas human beings are simultaneously biologic organisms, psychologic selves, behaving animals, and members of social systems, we lack a comprehensive set of general "laws" that include the models described here as biologic, psychologic, behavioral, and social. Failing that, we must come to terms with the following observations:

1. *No model offers a complete explanation for the phenomena to which it addresses itself.* Each model by its very definition ignores a universe of phenomena that are important in the patient's life and function. In limited cases, nevertheless, a single conceptual model will suffice to explain the disorder and provide treatment. The hallucination of a patient suffering from bromidism may indeed reflect prior personal experience, but the patient can be restored to health by detoxification with no attention paid to the psychologic content of his hallucinations.

2. *Any two conceptual models may offer alternative explanations for the same behavioral events.* For example, the psychodynamic clinician may argue that the relief of phobias obtained by "reciprocal inhibition" is in fact a "transference cure" — that is, it is the relation between the therapist and patient, rather than the technics of relaxation and desensitization to fear, that accounts for the beneficial outcome. Contrariwise, the behaviorist may contend that the psychotherapist is employing reinforcement methods rather than psychodynamic principles in shaping the behavior of his patient.

3. *In applying more than one conceptual model in treating a given patient, we must recognize the possibility of apparent contradictions.* In other words, pieces borrowed from more than one theory for simultaneous use in a given case may be orthogonal to one another. As a result, we give our patient mixed messages. For example, a schizophrenic patient may simultaneously be given medication (which implies a biologic basis for his disorder), be offered psychotherapy (which implies that past experience accounts for present dysfunction), be a member of a therapeutic community (which implies that he must control the behavior that distresses others), and be subject to a "token economy" in which healthy behavior is rewarded by tokens that bring special privileges.

Comparable Dilemmas in Other Fields

The importance of attention to each of the levels at which the patient functions is as important in other areas of medicine as it is in psychiatry. The patient with chronic rheumatoid arthritis suffers from a biologic disorder for which a number of nonspecific pharmacologic remedies exist. Whether the patient ends bedridden with ankylosed limbs may depend on how faithful he is in carrying out the prescribed exercises. This in turn will depend on his motivation, his relations to his physician and family, and the availability of facilities for physical therapy in the community. Disagreement between physicians about treatment is not unique to psychiatry. The patient with a bleeding peptic ulcer who consults a surgeon is more likely to have a gastrectomy than the one who consults an internist; a carcinoma of the breast will be treated by simple mastectomy in one hospital and by radical mastectomy in another.

The conceptual problems described in this chapter reflect limitations in our understanding of human behavior. In good clinical practice, a clinician will employ several conceptual models with the knowledge that all reflect some aspect of truth but all are incomplete versions of truth. The test of clinical skill is the assemblage of an appropriate mix for a particular case. To accomplish this best, the clinician should be explicit about the models that he employs in assessing a case and about the principles upon which he bases his treatment.

SUMMARY

This chapter attempts to make explicit the conceptual models that are implicit in clinical psychiatric practice. By doing so, the decision-making process in mental health practice can become more rational, a broader range of treatment modalities should be made available, and communication between clinicians should be enhanced.

The four conceptual models commonly used in clinical practice are the biologic, psychologic, behavioral, and social. Clinicians implicitly use one or a combination of models in evaluating and treating the patient by the process of clinical judgement. Some of the variables that determine the choice of conceptual models include the ideology of the therapist, the diagnosis, the effectiveness of available treatments, social class and other related variables, available services, and the immediacy of the social situation. The test of clinical skill is the assemblage of an appropriate mix for a particular case.

REFERENCES

1. Slater E, Roth M: *Clinical Psychiatry.* Third edition. Baltimore. Williams and Wilkins Company, 1969.
2. Kiloh LG, Garside RF: The independence of neurotic depression and endogenous depression. *Br J Psychiatry 109*:451–463, 1963.

3. Rosenthal SH, Gudeman JE: The endogenous depressive pattern: an empirical investigation. *Arch Gen Psychiatry 16*:241-249, 1967.

4. Semrad EV: *Teaching Psychotherapy of Psychotic Patients: Supervision of beginning residents in the "clinical approach."* New York, Grune and Stratton, 1969.

5. Alexander F, French TM: *Psychoanalytic Therapy: Principles and application.* New York, Ronald Press Company, 1946.

6. Deutsch H: Absence of grief. *Psychoanal Q 6*: 12-22, 1937.

7. Freud S: *Mourning and melancholia (1917), Collected Papers.* Vol 4. New York, Basic Books, Inc, 1959, pp. 152-170.

8. Urban HB, Ford DH: *Behavior therapy, Comprehensive Textbook of Psychiatry.* Edited by AM Freedman, HI Kaplan. Baltimore, Williams and Wilkins Company, 1967, pp. 1217-1224.

9. Liberman RP, Raskin DE: Depression: a behavioral formulation. *Arch Gen Psychiatry 24*: 515-523, 1971.

10. Liberman R: Behavioral approaches to family and couple therapy. *Am J Orthopsychiatry 40*: 106-118, 1970.

11. Lazarus AA: Learning theory and the treatment of depression. *Behav Res Ther 6*:83-89, 1968.

12. Thomas CS, Bergen BJ: Social psychiatric view of psychological misfunction and role of psychiatry in social change. *Arch Gen Psychiatry 12*:539-544, 1965.

13. Weiss RJ, Bergen BJ: Social supports and the reduction of psychiatric disability. *Psychiatry 31*:107-115, 1968.

14. Coleman JV: Social factors influencing the development and containment of psychiatric symptoms, *Mental Illness and Social Processes.* Edited by TJ Scheff. New York, Harper and Row, 1967, pp. 58-68.

15. *Idem:* Adaptive integration of psychiatric symptoms in ego regulation. *Arch Gen Psychiatry 24*:17-21, 1971.

16. Armor DJ, Klerman GL: Psychiatric treatment orientations and professional ideology. *J Health Soc Behav 9*:243-255, 1968.

17. Sharaf MR, Levinson DJ: Patterns of ideology and role definition among psychiatric residents. *The Patient and the Mental Hospital.* Edited by M Greenblatt, DJ Levinson, RH Williams. Glencoe, Illinois, Free Press, 1957, pp. 263-285.

18. Gilbert DC, Levinson DJ: Ideology, personality, and institutional policy in the mental hospital. *J Abnorm Soc Psychol 53*:263-271, 1956.

19. MacIver J, Redlich FC: Patterns of psychiatric practice. *Am J Psychiatry 115*:692-697, 1959.

20. Ehrlich D, Sabshin M: A study of sociotherapeutically oriented psychiatrists. *Am J Orthopsychiatry 34*:469-480, 1964.

21. Wender PH: The role of genetics in the etiology of the schizophrenias. *Am J Orthopsychiatry 39*:447-458, 1969.

22. Winokur G, Clayton PJ, Reich T: *Manic Depressive Illness.* St. Louis, CV Mosby Company, 1969.

23. Feighner JP, Robins E, Guze SB, et al.: Diagnostic criteria for use in psychiatric research. *Arch Gen Psychiatry 26*:57-63, 1972.

24. Truax CB, Carkhuff RR: *Toward Effective Counseling and Psychotherapy: Training and practice.* Chicago, Aldine-Atherton, Inc. 1967.
25. Meltzoff J, Kornreich M: Research in Psychotherapy. Chicago, Aldine-Atherton, Inc. 1970.
26. Hollingshead AB, Redlich FC: *Social Class and Mental Illness: A community study.* New York, John Wiley and Sons, 1958.
27. Lief HI, Lief VF, Warren CO et al.: Low dropout rate in a psychiatric clinic: special reference to psychotherapy and social class. *Arch Gen Psychiatry 5*:200–211, 1961.
28. Schaffer L, Myers JK: Psychotherapy and social stratification: an empirical study of practice in a psychiatric outpatient clinic. *Psychiatry 17*:83–93, 1954.
29. Myers JK, Schaffer L: Social stratification and psychiatric practice: a study of an out-patient clinic. *Am Social Rev 19*:307–310, 1954.
30. Overall B, Aronson H: Expectations of psychotherapy in patients of lower socioeconomic class. *Am J Orthopsychiatry 33*:421–430, 1963.
31. Levinson DJ, Merrifield J, Berg K: Becoming a patient. *Arch Gen Psychiatry 17*:385–406, 1967.
32. Heine RW, Trosman H: Initial expectations of the doctor-patient interaction as a factor in continuance in psychotherapy. *Psychiatry 23*: 275–278, 1960.
33. Schildkraut JJ: The catecholamine hypothesis of affective disorders: a review of supporting evidence. *Am J Psychiatry 122*:509–522, 1965.
34. Schildkraut JJ, Kety SS: Biogenic amines and emotion. *Science 156*:21–30, 1967.
35. Caudill WA: *The Psychiatric Hospital as a Small Society.* Cambridge, Harvard University Press, 1958.
36. Stanton AH, Schwartz MS: *The Mental Hospital: A study of institutional participation in psychiatric illness and treatment.* New York, Basic Books, Inc., 1954.
37. Caplan G, Caplan RB: Development of community psychiatry concepts, *Comprehensive Textbook of Psychiatry.* Edited by AM Freedman, HI Kaplan. Baltimore, Williams and Wilkins Company, 1967, pp. 1499–1516.
38. Marmor J: Dynamic psychotherapy and behavior therapy: are they irreconcilable? *Arch Gen Psychiatry 24*:22–28, 1971.
39. Marks IM, Gelder MG: Common ground between behaviour therapy and psychodynamic methods. *Br J Med Psychol 39*:11–23, 1966.
40. Miller NE: Learning of visceral and glandular responses. *Science 163*:434–445, 1969.

2

an interview

for community settings

Clinicians initially learn the techniques of interviewing and evaluation by collecting and recording large numbers of observations from patients whom they see over an extended period of time. The data are then organized in some fashion such as chief complaint, present illness, family history, developmental history, sexual history, occupational history, medical history, and mental status examination. Finally, the clinician sorts out symptoms, themes, and processes in order to establish a diagnosis and formulation. The opportunity for this kind of intensive study is provided by inpatient units where patients stay for a long enough period of time and by psychotherapy clinics where patients are stable enough to return for several visits.

This chapter is adapted from Aaron Lazare, "The Psychiatric Examination in the Walk-In Clinic: Hypothesis Generation and Hypothesis Testing," *Archives of General Psychiatry* (in press). Copyright 1975 by *Archives of General Psychiatry* and American Medical Association.

As clinicians gain experience over months and years, they begin to take shortcuts. Sensing where the "pay dirt" is, they ignore extraneous information while focusing their energies on the elicitation of data that are apt to make a difference in clinical management. This improvement in efficiency becomes necessary because they soon are expected to make more rapid decisions in order to provide competent care for more patients per unit time.

What clinicians have done in developing their skills is to change strategies for diagnosis and care formulation from the collection and assimilation of large amounts of data to the generation and testing of various hypotheses. Using this new approach, they consider a limited number of possibilities based on critical observations usually made early in the interview. They then proceed to elicit specific data to confirm or refute the hypothesis under consideration rather than to obtain a complete history. For the expert clinician, the probability that the correct diagnosis or formulation will be found among the early hypotheses is quite high.[1-3]*

In the community, in walk-in clinics, emergency psychiatric services, health maintenance organizations, and the ambulatory services of community mental health centers, where a primary goal is rapid assessment and decision making, it is obviously difficult to collect and to assimilate large amounts of data. Yet clinicians must decide within a limited amount of time whether or not a patient is suicidal, is in need of hospitalization, needs psychotropic agents, can be helped in a few sessions, needs an extended diagnostic evaluation, or may leave with no further care. The danger is always present that incomplete data will result in incorrect decisions.

In this chapter, we shall attempt to formulate a hypothesis-generating and testing approach for the initial psychiatric examination in the community and related settings. Sixteen hypotheses that we and our colleagues have found useful in organizing clinical data will be described. We shall attempt to show that this approach (1) helps the clinician make efficient use of limited time in attempting to be comprehensive, (2) guards the clinician from coming to premature closure in the collection of data, and (3) provides a stimulus for the exploration of relevant but neglected clinical questions.

In considering the interview as hypothesis generation and testing, the focus is on the collection and organization of data. Three important dimensions of the psychiatric examination that will *not*

*Superscript numbers in this chapter refer to numbered references at end of this chapter.

be discussed are (1) the patient's goals and requests (see Chapter 3); (2) the therapeutic aspects of the clinician–patient interaction, including the negotiation of goals and requests, which hopefully occur even before a specific treatment plan is formulated; and (3) the techniques necessary to elicit relevant data.

A MULTIDIMENSIONAL APPROACH

The hypotheses to be considered and the clinical methods needed to test them depend on a theoretical framework. We shall, therefore, review the approach that we have found useful. This approach and its clinical implications are discussed more fully in Chapter 1.

Although "human beings are simultaneously biological organisms, psychological selves, behaving animals, and members of social systems," there is a lack of a theory of human behavior that satisfactorily integrates these four dimensions. Attempts by psychoanalysts, behaviorists, or general system theorists to describe a comprehensive theory of human behavior are either too cumbersome or not adequately inclusive. Clinicians, in the absence of such a comprehensive theory, implicitly use one or a combination of models that include the psychologic, social, biologic, and behavioral. These models may be thought of as different lenses through which one can observe a single object. Each lens has its own value and each has its own limitations.

The choice of conceptual approach in clinical practice has serious implications since it may determine the method by which one collects data, the data that are considered relevant, and the treatment that is most appropriate. For example, a clinician using a psychologic approach may examine the psychologic meaning of the precipitating event in order to understand the issues that have led to the depression. A clinician using a social approach to examine the same patient may determine how the disruption of the social matrix led to the patient's depression. Hopefully, there will be some way of reestablishing some social equilibrium. Using a biologic approach, the clinician will inquire into the signs and symptoms of a unipolar or bipolar depression, previous episodes of depression, and family history of depressive illness, in the hopes of diagnosing a syndrome for which there is a somatic treatment. Using a behavioral approach, the clinician will elicit the undesired behaviors together with their antecedent and reinforcing conditions in the hopes of positively reinforcing normal behavior or extinguishing depressive behavior.

In clinical practice, the use of one or a combination of the four conceptual models is implicitly determined by many variables. These include the ideology of the therapist, the diagnosis, the responsiveness of the symptoms to somatic treatment, the treatment resources, the social class of the patient, and other personal attributes such as verbal intelligence, psychological mindedness, young adult age, psychological strengths, likability, and attractiveness.[5]

Clinicians are sometimes unaware of how these variables influence their clinical judgment. When this happens, they run the risk of dealing with diffuse and incomplete data, an approach that may be inappropriately termed "eclectic."[6]

In the examination of the patient in or from the community for whom various conceptual frameworks are often relevant, the pitfalls described above can be minimized by simultaneously formulating the problem from psychologic, social, biologic, and behavioral perspectives. This means that hypotheses from all four theoretical frameworks are considered. In this way the chances of making the appropriate clinical mix yielding the optimal therapeutic gain will be enhanced.[4,7,8,9]

HYPOTHESES (HYPOTHESIZED PARTIAL FORMULATIONS)

The clinician brings to the interview partial formulations based on previous experience. A formulation is defined here as a concept that organizes, explains, or makes clinical sense out of large amounts of data and influences the treatment decision. These concepts include clinical syndromes such as schizophrenia, personality styles such as the hysterical personality, social conditions such as social isolation, and even symptoms such as suicidal behavior. These concepts may be "apples and oranges," but they do represent clusters of information that clinicians find useful in understanding patients. In Weisman's terms, "This is the nature of communication between people—to operate on many levels at once with different words, different objects, and different meanings."[10] These concepts are partial formulations because any one alone is insufficient to provide adequate understanding of any given patient. In the process of bringing these partial formulations to the interview for consideration, they become hypotheses to be tested.

Clinicians, by thinking in terms of hypotheses, keep themselves from being bombarded or overloaded with large amounts of unstructured data, an experience shared by all beginners. Each new

observation can now be considered in terms of its relevance to a limited number of hypotheses under consideration instead of being one out of thousands of possible facts.[11]

Two problems immediately arise in applying this approach to the psychiatric examination. The first is that in considering a few hypotheses usually generated early in the interview, the clinician may come to premature closure, thereby ignoring more relevant hypotheses. The second is that, given the rich and varied data that can be collected, there must be thousands of possible hypotheses or ways of organizing data. A solution to both problems would be the development of a manageable list of hypothesized partial formulations based on current knowledge which would organize most of the observations that might relate to decision making. The entire range of hypotheses could then be considered, at least briefly, during each interview. The composition of such a list might vary with the clinical setting and would undoubtedly change with advances in the field.

This chapter will propose 16 hypotheses that we and our colleagues have found useful in evaluating and treating patients in the community and related settings. They are organized under four major headings: "Psychologic," "Social," "Biologic," and "Behavioral" (according to the conceptual approach whose theory and methods generate, confirm, or refute the hypothesis). These hypothesized partial formulations are intended to become neither decision trees nor a complete list of diagnoses. Rather, they are intended to assist in the clinical understanding of the vast majority of patients so that decisions can more effectively be made.

There is some overlap between various partial formulations since they may explain similar observations from different perspectives. For instance, calling a patient schizoid (psychologic) or socially isolated (social) may be describing some of the same phenomena from different perspectives.

For any given patient, several partial formulations will be necessary to approach "complete understanding." For example, knowing that a patient is suffering from unresolved grief tells us a great deal. Add to this partial formulation the knowledge of an obsessional personality style, the ego's incapacity to bear painful affective states, relative social isolation, and a behavioral system that punishes grieving behavior. These additional partial formulations provide the clinician with considerably more power to understand and to treat the patient.

I. Psychologic Hypotheses

1. *Knowledge of the patient's **personality style** explains in part why he has come for treatment.*

Knowledge of the personality style may be important in understanding the patient's psychological vulnerabilities and therefore the meaning of the stress or precipitating event. It may also predict the defensive posture that the patient will employ to keep the clinician from reaching the important psychological issues surrounding the current problem.[12-15] Armed with this knowledge, the clinician can avoid the patient's diversionary tactics and more effectively find the heart of the matter. This hypothesis, with its potential for making sense from large amounts of data, can often be inferred from a relatively small number of observations obtained early in the interview.

2. *Knowledge of the **precipitating event** and its dynamic meaning explains in part why the patient has come for treatment.*

It is essential to learn the stress or precipitating event (when present) that precedes the onset of symptoms. At least as important is the psychological meaning of this event. Does the event mean to the patient that he is now hopeless, weak, powerless, out of control, destructive, bad, a failure, unreal, or unloved? Does it mean to him that he is attacked, penetrated, violated, damaged, overwhelmed, smothered, ridiculed, or cheated?[16-19] Is the precipitating event evidence of a recurrent neurotic theme? Knowing the psychological meaning of the event improves rapport because the patient now believes the clinician really appreciates what is happening. At least as important, the clinician may know with considerable specificity the psychological work that needs to be done.

3. *The patient's problem can be understood in part as a manifestation of **unresolved grief**.*

This hypothesis is a variation of the previous one when it is determined, for instance, that the symptoms followed a loss that the patient inadequately mourned. The grief hypothesis, however,

is worth considering separately for several reasons: (1) The symptom picture may not follow a discrete stress but may occur after an anniversary of a loss, after a holiday, or after a minor event symbolizing the loss. (2) The symptom picture of unresolved grief represents a relatively clear-cut clinical syndrome.[20] (3) Specific methods must be employed to elicit the necessary observations to confirm or refute the hypothesis. (4) A relatively high incidence of patients are seen for whom unresolved grief is an important issue.

> **4.** *The patient's problem can be understood in part as a developmental crisis.*

When it is difficult to understand the patient's presentation as a reaction to a discrete event or as a manifestation of unresolved grief, the problem may be better understood as part of a developmental crisis. Using this approach, the clinician considers what series of issues the patient may be suffering from at this stage of development. For instance, a 50-year-old female may well be simultaneously struggling with menopause, children leaving home, strains in the marital relationship, and the death of a parent. With the developmental crisis hypothesis in mind, the clinician can elicit specific historical data that may clarify the clinical problem.[21, 22]

> **5.** *The patient's problem can be understood in part in terms of ego functioning and related psychodynamic issues.*

There are many subconcepts or ways of organizing the data of ego assessment and related psychodynamic issues. These include recurrent neurotic themes, meaning of neurotic symptoms, predominant defense mechanisms, overall defensive success, reality testing, sense of reality, judgment, thought processes, tolerance to stress, capacity to bear affects, impulse control, patterns of regression, autonomous functioning, synthetic functioning, conflict-free areas, libidinal fixation, object relations, sexual identification, superego severity and integration, and psychological mindedness. A clinician using a psychodynamic approach usually chooses a few of these overlapping concepts to help explain the patient's problem and to plan treatment. Confirmation of the ego assessment hypothesis often requires data from many sources, including developmental history, dreams, associations, and transference reactions.[23-25]

II. Social Hypotheses

6. Cultural factors *explain in part the patient's problem and his reasons for seeking treatment.*

It is important to consider to what degree cultural factors influence perceptions, beliefs, values, behavioral norms, and expectations that give clues as to the choice, expression, and seriousness of symptomatology. Cultural factors also influence the choice of and attitudes toward treatment and even the basic communicative processes between clinician and patient.[26–31]

7. *The patient's problem can be understood in part in terms of a* **change in the social space.**

The social space (social network) consists of all relevent people (and animals) in the patient's life—at home, with friends, at school, and on the job. The clinical presentation can often be understood in terms of a disruption or impending disruption of the social space that had previously supported the patient. To explore this hypothesis, the patient may be asked to list and to describe briefly all the important people in his life. By listening for the order in which people are listed, for the associated affective responses, and for the omissions of important people, the clinical picture often falls into place. The recovery process will depend in large part on the availability of important relationships.[31–35]

8. Social isolation *explains in part the patient's problem.*

For many patients who present to a walk-in clinic, the paucity of their social contacts may explain what they ask for and what they need from the clinician.[36] They often make modest requests, perhaps a prescription refill or someone to speak with for a few minutes. The social isolation may be characterological in origin or it may be the result of social transition such as a recent move. Shuval has shown that social transition is a cause for presentation to medical clinics in Israel.[37] This hypothesis is tested only by specific inquiry into the patient's social space.

9. *The patient's problem can be understood in part as a* **social communication.**

The symptom or even the clinic visit can be understood as an attempt to influence or to communicate something to some person, social group, or institution. This hypothesis, like the one above, can be determined by reviewing the people or groups in the patient's life space. The questions are who wants what from whom and who is doing what to whom? Sometimes the communication can be discerned by watching the patient with a relative in the waiting room or at a family conference. The communication may or may not be conscious.[38-43]

> *10. The patient's problem can be understood in part in terms of its **social impact**, including suicide or violence.*

The importance of this hypothesis is self-evident. Once it is confirmed that the patient is suicidal, violent, or in danger of harming others, the clinician then calls forth a new body of knowledge to explore the seriousness of the aggression, etiology, treatability, and follow-up.

III. Biologic Hypotheses

> *11. The patient's problem can be understood in part as an **affective disorder** (unipolar or bipolar).[44-46]*

This hypothesis should be considered because of its relatively high incidence, its treatability, the dangers inherent in the clinical course when rigorous treatment is delayed, and the important differential diagnosis of syndromes that present as affective disorders. Although psychologic, social, and behavioral considerations are essential in the understanding and management of these patients, affective disorder is listed as biologic since the hypothesis is usually established by the method of the biologic approach—observations of signs and symptoms through time. In addition, there are important somatic treatments for these disorders.

> *12. The patient is suffering in part from **schizophrenia**.[45-48]*

This hypothesis, like the previous one, should be considered because of its frequency, its treatability, the dangers inherent in its clinical course when treatment is delayed, and the differential diagnoses of syndromes that present in this manner. Although the hypothesis is usually established by the biologic method, psychodynamic, social, and behavioral considerations are essential in the understanding and management of these patients.

13. *The patient's problem can be understood in part as an* **organic disease.**

It is useful to divide this hypothesis into conditions that present with and without impairments of the sensorium. The latter group is most apt to be overlooked. The clinician should consider a differential diagnosis that includes organic illness even in the presence of a clear sensorium when he observes psychotic thinking, mania, depression, anxiety, impotence, eneuresis, syncope, amnesia, pain, and various sensory and motor disturbances.

14. *The patient is suffering in part from* **alcohol** *or* **drug abuse.**

This hypothesis deserves separate consideration since (1) its occurrence is common; (2) patients are reluctant to acknowledge their abuse of alcohol and drugs; (3) health professionals, because of hostile feelings toward many of these patients, may overlook the problem; (4) the abuse of these agents, aside from their complex causes, sets in motion a series of medical, social, and psychological problems that may require special therapeutic techniques.

15. *The patient's problem can be understood in part in terms of symptoms responsive to* **psychotropic agents.**

The separate consideration of psychotropic agents ensures that an important treatment possibility is not overlooked.

IV. Behavioral Hypotheses

16. *The patient's problem can be understood in part in* **behavioral** *terms.*

For each patient, the clinician should consider whether an understanding of the undesired behaviors together with their antecedent and reinforcing events will lead to a plan of treatment. In addition, it should be considered whether there already exist specific treatment programs for these behaviors.[49, 50]

THE DYNAMICS OF HYPOTHESIS GENERATION AND TESTING

Hypothesis generation and testing can be thought of as a three-step mental process repeated many times throughout the interview by which the clinician (1) collects data (makes observations); (2) generates, confirms, and refutes hypotheses on the basis of the data collected; and (3) employs clinical methods or strategies to elicit further data that will generate new hypotheses and confirm or refute old ones.

Data Collection

The observations or data that lead to hypothesis generation, confirmation, and refutation may come from (1) outside the patient (previous records, clinic face sheet, information from the family); (2) the patient's biographical reconstructions; (3) the mental status examination (behavior observations made during the interview); (4) the physical examination and laboratory data; and (5) psychodynamic material including dreams, fantasies, memories, associations, recurrent themes, and transference and countertransference reactions; and (6) social interactions in waiting rooms, family conferences, homes, or neighborhoods.

What there is to observe is a result of the clinician's methods, the patient's pathology, and other dimensions of the clinical situation such as the size of the room, the position of the chairs, the duration of the wait, the time of day, etc. The clinician's ability to perceive the observations depends on what is thought to be important and on the ability to observe.

Hypothesis Generation and Testing

Although the clinician can briefly consider all the hypotheses on the list, it is usually possible to explore only a few in depth. The selection of these few is best determined by several criteria.

1. One considers hypotheses that are most probable on the basis of available data. For example, fastidious dress may lead to consideration of an obsessional style; recurrent presentations on the same date may lead to consideration of unresolved grief.
2. One considers those hypotheses that are most serious even though they may not be highly probable. These include suicide intent, organic brain disease, and schizophrenia.
3. One gives special consideration to those hypotheses that have a high probability of being reversed with treatment such as primary affective disorders, unresolved grief, and acute brain syndromes.
4. One considers those hypotheses for which there are treatment resources. For example, if psychotherapy time is available, one explores various ego functions to determine whether the patient is a candidate for this treatment.

5. One considers those hypotheses that the patient believes are relevant. The patient is often right and, if he is wrong, it will be important that he know his concerns have been taken seriously.

Which hypotheses the clinicians test depends not only on the priorities listed above but on their awareness of the range of hypotheses to be tested and on their ability to relate specific data to the formation, refutation, and confirmation of hypotheses. For instance, clinicians must know that delusions may be part of schizophrenia, affective disorders, or organic brain disease if this symptom is to alert them to test these hypotheses.

Strategies (methods)

After the clinician generates several hypotheses on the basis of the available observations, he develops a strategy to test these hypotheses. To do this the clinician must know what further data are required to confirm or to refute any given hypothesis. He then sets out to collect this data by various methods such as direct questioning, sitting in silence, employing the associative anamnestic technique, encouraging free associations, speaking to the family, testing the patient's memory, paying attention to his own subjective responses, stressing the patient, using sodium amytal, or evaluating the response of a trial medication. Many of these methods can be traced to the four basic conceptual frameworks previously described. The effectiveness of the method will depend on choosing the proper one for the particular hypothesis, the skill of the clinician, and the responsiveness of the patient. Particular methods may have to be withheld if they are antitherapeutic. For example, the stress of extended silence may yield useful data but impair the treatment relationship.

Conduct of the Interview

In conducting the interview, the clinician proceeds in the usual manner by first asking the patient what brought him to the clinic and then elaborating the events, symptoms, and issues of the present illness. It is neither necessary nor desirable to ask questions systematically about each successive hypothesis. Such a procedure would reduce the interview to a disjointed interrogation. The clinician, in gathering the relevant information, is as active and directive as necessary for diagnostic completeness. At the same time, he remains as nondirective as possible so as to preserve the free flow of the patient's thoughts.

Many of the hypotheses can be tested without the clinician's interfering at all with the flow of the interview. For instance, one can refute with relative certainty the idea that the patient is suffering from an organic illness with disturbed sensorium when the presentation is psychologically understandable, when there is no schizophreniclike or severe affective symptomatology, when the patient appears physically well, and when there is no evidence of intellectual impairment as inferred from the patient's presentation of the history. All of these observations can be made with little or no verbal activity on the part of the clinician. Much of the evidence about personality style and ego assessment is derived in a similar fashion. Even when hypotheses require direct questioning for their confirmation, the questions can often become a part of the natural flow of the interview.

We have found it very useful to review the complete list of hypotheses in two specific circumstances during the clinical examination. The first is when the hypotheses that spontaneously arise during the first 10 to 15 minutes of the interview fail to make clinical sense out of the data. The review becomes a source of new ideas, new approaches, and new meanings for previously discarded observations. The second circumstance in which we review all the hypotheses is 5 to 10 minutes prior to completing each interview. This ensures that all the major diagnostic and therapeutic possibilities have been considered. We have been surprised at how often such an approach leads to the elicitation of data that significantly supplements the working case formulation. For example, during a 30-minute interview, data were elicited that led to the following partial formulation: The patient, a 38-year-old Roman Catholic female, reported mild depressive symptomatology beginning 12 months ago when she divorced her alcoholic husband. She had considerable ambivalence about the decision, she was now in a situation of relative social isolation, and she was feeling guilty about the possibility of renewed heterosexual contacts. These explanations for her clinical condition combining psychologic, social, and biologic hypotheses "felt right." Before completing the interview, the entire list of hypotheses was reviewed to ensure at least brief consideration of each. After pondering the unresolved grief hypothesis, the patient was asked whether anyone important to her had died. She immediately burst into tears as she told of her father-in-law's death 6 months before. This man, she explained, was a source of constant support to her. He shopped for her, listened to her troubles, and cared for her "more than my own husband." His relationship to her never faltered, even after the divorce. With his death there seemed to be no one to support her in her grief over this seemingly distant relationship. The patient then recalled that she had been depressed for the 6 months since her father-in-law's death, not for the 12 months since the divorce. Without reviewing the hypotheses, this added partial formulation, given the pressure of time, might have been omitted.

Mental health professionals have set for themselves the task of delivering care in clinical settings requiring rapid assessment and decision making. Toward this end, enormous energy has been expended to develop complex delivery systems employing a wide variety of mental health professionals. Despite this effort, the systems often deliver empty packages.

In order to improve the quality of care, one of our tasks will be the reorganization of clinical knowledge acquired from in-depth work with patients and its reapplication and transmission to new clinical settings. The hypothesis-generation and testing approach together with the development of a closed system of hypotheses is offered as one such way of reorganizing ideas. This approach is not intended to oversimplify the enormously complex clinical process. Rather, it analyzes and makes explicit this process so that learning may be facilitated.

In our own clinical areas, we have begun teaching the community interview by this approach. In doing so, we have found that the language of hypothesis testing raises several important questions whose relevance is not limited to a particular clinical setting:

1. For a particular setting, what is the best way to organize data into hypotheses that are intellectually manageable and clinically useful?
2. What clinical observations should lead to the generation of a given hypothesis?
3. Conversely, what hypotheses should be generated by a given observation?
4. What data are necessary to confirm or refute any given hypothesis?
5. What methods or strategies may be employed to collect data necessary for the confirmation and refutation of a given hypothesis?

These questions are seldom asked or answered in textbooks of nursing, psychiatry, psychology, or social work. Clinicians, nevertheless, deal with them implicitly in deciding what to look for, how to look for it, and when to look for it. Such skills and processes are the heart of clinical practice. We learn them from teachers and from clinical experience, and we pass them on by the oral tradition. It is hoped that by making these processes explicit, much of what is now called clinical skill or intuition can more effectively be communicated by the written word. Our ability to learn from each other will then be enhanced, and what we believe to be true can more easily become subject to validation.

REFERENCES

1. Sandifer MG, Hordern A, Green LM: The psychiatric interview: the impact of the first three minutes. *Amer J Psychiat 126*:968–973, 1970.
2. Pittenger RE, Hockett CF, Danehy JJ: *The First Five Minutes.* Ithaca, New York, Paul Martineau, 1960.
3. Gauron EF, Dickinson JK: Diagnostic decision making in psychiatry: (1) information usage. *Arch Gen Psychiat 14*:225–232, 1966.
4. Lazare A: Hidden conceptual models in clinical psychiatry. *New Eng J Med 288*:345–351, 1973.
5. Levinson DJ, Merrifield J, Berg K: Becoming a patient. *Arch Gen Psychiat 17*:385–406, 1967.
6. Simon RM: On eclecticism. *Amer J Psychiat 131*:135–139, 1974.
7. Freedman DX, Gordon RP: Psychiatry under siege: attacks from without. *Psychiatric Annals 3*:10–34, November 1973.
8. Havens LL: Clinical methods in psychiatry. *Internat J Psychiat 10*:7–28, 1972.
9. Havens LL: *Approaches to the Mind.* Boston, Little, Brown and Company, 1973.
10. Weisman AD: The psychodynamic formulation of conflict. *Arch Gen Psychiat 1*:288–309, 1959.
11. Elstein AS, Kagan N, Shulman LS, Jason H, Loupe MJ: Methods and theory in the study of medical inquiry. *J Med Educ 47*:85–92, 1972.
12. Shapiro D: *Neurotic Styles.* New York, Basic Books, Inc., 1965.
13. Kahana RJ, Bibring GL: Personality types in medical management, *Psychiatry and Medical Practice in a General Hospital.* Edited by N. Zinberg, New York, International Universities Press, 1964.
14. Lazare A: The hysterical character in psychoanalytic theory: evolution and confusion. *Arch Gen Psychiat 25*:131–137, 1971.
15. Lazare A, Klerman GL, Armor D: Oral, obsessive and hysterical personality patterns: replication of factor analysis in an independent sample. *J Psychiat Res 7*:275–290, 1970.
16. Harris MR, Kalis BL, Freeman EH: Precipitating stress: an approach to brief therapy. *Amer J Psychother 17*:465–471, 1963.
17. Kalis BL, Harris MR, Prestwood AR, Freedman EH: Precipitating stress as a focus in psychotherapy. *Arch Gen Psychiat 5*:219, 1961.
18. Coleman JV: Aims and conduct of psychotherapy. *Arch Gen Psychiat 18*:1–6, 1968.
19. Bibring E: The mechanism of depression, in Greenacre P (ed): *Affective Disorders.* New York, International Universities Press, 1953.
20. Parkes CM: *Bereavement: Studies of Grief in Adult Life.* New York, International Universities Press, 1972.

21. Erikson EH: *Childhood and Society.* New York, W. W. Norton & Company, Inc., 1950.
22. Schwartz LH, Schwartz JL: *The Psychodynamics of Patient Care.* Englewood Cliffs, N.J., Prentice-Hall, Inc., 1972.
23. Bellak L, Hurvich M, Gediman HK: *Ego Functions in Schizophrenics, Neurotics, and Normals.* New York, John Wiley & Sons, 1973.
24. Prelinger E, Zimet CN: *An Ego-Psychological Approach to Character Assessment.* London, The Free Press of Glencoe, Collier-Macmillan Limited, 1964.
25. Vaillant GE: Theoretical hierarchy of adaptive ego mechanisms. A 30-year follow-up of 30 men selected for psychological health. *Arch Gen Psychiat 24*:107–118, 1971.
26. Mechanic D: Social psychological factors affecting the presentation of bodily complaints. *New Eng J Med 286*:1132, 1972.
27. Wittkower ED, Dubreuil G: Psychocultural stress in relation to mental illness. *Soc Sci Med 7*:691–704, 1973.
28. Fox R: Illness, *International Encyclopedia of the Social Sciences,* Vol. 7. Edited by D Sills. New York, Macmillan, 1968.
29. Zola I: Culture and symptoms. *Amer Soc Rev 31*:615, 1966.
30. Nader L, Maretzki T (eds): *Cultural Illness and Health: Essays in Human Adaptation.* Washington, D.C., American Anthropological Association, 1973.
31. Tseng WH: The development of psychiatric concepts in traditional Chinese medicine. *Arch Gen Psychiat 29*:569–575, 1973.
32. Thomas CS, Bergen BJ: Social psychiatric view of psychological misfunction and role of psychiatry in social change. *Arch Gen Psychiat 12*:539–544, 1965.
33. Rahe RH: Subjects' recent life changes and their near-future illness susceptibility in Lipowski ZJ (ed): *Advances in Psychosomatic Medicine,* Vol. 8. Basil, Switzerland, S. Karger, 1972.
34. Coleman JV: Social factors influencing the development and containment of psychiatric symptoms, edited by TJ Scheff. *Mental Illness and Social Processes.* New York, Harper and Row, 1967.
35. Coleman JV: Adaptive integration of psychiatric symptoms in ego regulation. *Arch Gen Psychiat 24*:17–21, 1971.
36. Dunham HW: Resolving competing hypotheses, *Social Psychology and Mental Health.* Edited by H Wechsler, L Solomon, and BM Kramer. New York, Holt, Rinehart and Winston, Inc., 1970.
37. Shuval JT: *Social Functions of Medical Practice: Doctor-Patient Relationships in Israel.* San Francisco, Jossey-Bass, 1970.
38. Ruesch J: General theory of communication in psychiatry, chap. 45, *American Handbook of Psychiatry,* Vol. 1. Edited by S Arieti. New York, Basic Books, Inc., 1959.
39. Spiegel R: Specific problems of communication in psychiatric conditions, chap. 46, *American Handbook of Psychiatry,* Vol. 1. Edited by S. Arieti. New York, Basic Books, Inc., 1959.
40. Ziegler RJ, Imboden JB: Contemporary conversion reactions. *Arch Gen Psychiat 6*:37–45, 1962.

41. Rabkin R: Conversion hysteria as social maladaptation. *Psychiatry* 27:349–363, 1964.
42. Berne E: *Games People Play*. New York, Grove Press, 1964.
43. Twaddle AC: The concepts of sick role and illness behavior, in Lipowski ZJ (ed): *Advances in Psychosomatic Medicine*, Vol. 8. Basil, Switzerland, S. Karger, 1972.
44. Winokur G, Clayton PJ, Reich T: *Manic Depressive Illness*. St. Louis, C. V. Mosby Co., 1969.
45. Feighner JP et al.: Diagnostic criteria for use in psychiatric research. *Arch Gen Psychiat* 26:57–63, 1972.
46. Woodruff RA, Goodwin DW, Guze SB: *Psychiatric Diagnoses*. New York, Oxford University Press, 1974.
47. Robins E, Guze SB: Establishment of diagnostic validity in psychiatric illness: its application to schizophrenia. *Amer J Psychiat* 126:983–987, 1970.
48. Wender PH: The role of genetics in the etiology of schizophrenia. *Amer J Orthopsychiat* 39:447–458, 1969.
49. Kanfer FH, Saslow G: Behavioral analysis: an alternative to diagnostic classification. *Arch Gen Psychiat* 12:529–538, 1965.
50. Franks CM (ed): *Behavior Therapy: Appraisal and Status*. New York, McGraw-Hill Book Company, 1969.

3

the customer approach
to patienthood

It is a frustrating and fatiguing experience to treat patients and teach personnel in community settings. Large numbers of patients want immediate help with a heterogeneous group of problems that do not easily lend themselves to official diagnostic categories or psychodynamic formulations. As a result, the clinician is always in danger of feeling drained and helpless. The psychotherapy clinic and the inpatient unit, in contrast, are able to screen their admissions for the proper number and kind of patients for whom they have developed treatment programs. There is at least some consensus as to the outpatient treatment of the neuroses and the hospital management of the psychoses.

Frustration with the numbers of patients and the kinds of problems they present may be dealt with in various nonproductive

This chapter is adapted from Aaron Lazare, Sherman Eisenthal, and Linda Wasserman, "The Customer Approach to Patienthood," *Archives of General Psychiatry,* 32:553–558. Copyright 1975 by the *Archives of General Psychiatry* and the American Medical Association; and from Aaron Lazare, Sherman Eisenthal, Linda Wasserman, and Thomas C. Harford, "Patient Requests in a Walk-In Clinic," *Comprehensive Psychiatry* 16 (5) Sept/Oct., 1975, pp. 467–77, reprinted with permission.

ways. The clinical settings may be relegated to second class status by limiting staffing and teaching allocations. The staff may cope by discouraging patients with excessive delays in the waiting period for treatment, by providing such brief therapy that it is inadequate therapy, or by playing "musical clinics," referring large numbers of patients to another facility, which, in turn, makes a further referral.

Despite the frustrations and fatigue, we have come to believe in the special importance of community settings as clinical services and as places to train personnel. Given this special importance, there is a need to reconceptualize and reorganize ideas around the walk-in patient so that patient care and staff morale are improved.

With the incentive of having to provide a meaningful training experience for the staff of a walk-in clinic of a general hospital,[1] * we set out to learn from patients what they wanted from the professionals who were there to serve them. Based on these observations and on subsequent research, we have been evolving the "customer approach to patienthood," which, we believe, is relevant to all mental health professionals.[2]

This approach is an attempt to conceptualize the initial interview as a process of negotiation between the clinician and the patient, taking the patient's request as a starting point. Most patients make one or more requests, many of which represent legitimate needs. These requests/needs include those for psychotherapy, psychiatric diagnoses and treatment, and many others. It is the clinician's task to elicit the patient's request, collect the relevant clinical data, and enter into a "negotiation." As a result, it is hoped that the patient will feel his perceived needs have been heard and responded to while the clinician will feel that he/she has been not only comprehensive but responsive to the patient. The negotiation should facilitate a relationship of mutual influence between clinician and patient to the benefit of both parties.

The initial interview as a negotiation is an elaboration of an idea described earlier by Levinson et al.[3] In this important paper, they contrast the "negotiated consensus" with both the "suitability" and the "diagnostic" approaches to patienthood. Using the "suitability approach," the clinic screens the patient to determine whether he fulfills the criteria to become "a good therapy case." Here the patient must have the credentials (young, verbal,

---

*Superscript numbers in this chapter refer to numbered references at end of this chapter.

motivated, etc.) to be offered the treatment the clinic is offering. Using the "diagnostic approach," the clinic determines on the basis of observable signs and symptoms whether or not the patient is suffering from a psychiatric illness. Many of the problems in delivering service in a walk-in clinic, we believe, result from an inappropriate use of suitability or diagnostic approaches.

In this chapter, we will describe the customer approach, its implementation, and its clinical importance. We will attempt to show that this approach to patienthood not only improves mental health care and patient satisfaction but also leads to improved staff morale.

IMPLEMENTATION OF THE CUSTOMER APPROACH

Patient Requests

The negotiation process between the patient (or prospective patient) and the clinician rests on the assumption that the patient has something in mind that he wants. To the surprise of many clinicians, the vast majority of patients who come to community clinics on their own volition know with considerable specificity how they would like the clinician to intervene on their behalf.

From our analysis of several hundred interviews we were able to classify patient requests into 14 categories.[2, 4] We have attempted to describe them below in terms which are meaningful to both clinician and patient and which lend themselves to therapeutic intervention.

Administrative request. The patient is seeking administrative or legal assistance from the clinic to help him with his current dilemma. The specific request may be to provide a disability evaluation, a draft deferment, a medical excuse to leave work, medical permission to return to work, permission to drive, admission to a hospital, or testimony in court. These powers are delegated by society to particular professionals or institutions. The power may be subsequently rescinded or, as in the case of therapeutic abortions, may no longer be necessary.

Advice. The patient wants guidance about what to do in personal or social matters. He may already have formed an opinion but now wants professional advice. He wants to know the "right" thing, the "best" thing, or the "wisest" thing to do. He may want the advice in order to have the clinician share the responsibility for a decision he is about to make.

Clarification. The patient wants help to put his feelings, thoughts, or behavior in some perspective. He does not want to be told what to do but would rather take an active role in the therapeutic process. Often the patient wants the help to be able to make a decision. He wants to understand; he wants to see his choices. The patient usually sees his problem as being acute and not a part of an ongoing neurotic pattern.

Community triage. The patient is requesting information as to where in his community he can find the help he needs. He sees the clinic as an available resource that has the necessary information.

Confession. The patient feels guilty about what he has said, thought, or done and hopes that by talking to the therapist he will feel better. Specifically, the patient wants to be forgiven. He hopes the clinician (authority figure) will see the misdeed as medical or psychological in origin and therefore not bad.

Control. The patient is feeling overwhelmed and out of control. He may fear hurting himself or someone else or going crazy. He is saying "Please take over. I can no longer manage."

Medical. The patient sees his problem as being physical in origin, like any other medical condition, as opposed to psychological or situational in origin. He often refers to his problem as "nerves" or as a "nervous condition." The patient, accordingly, hopes for a medical kind of treatment such as pills, ECT, hospitalization, or medical advice. He expects to take a passive role in the treatment.

Psychological expertise. The patient believes that the source of his problem is psychological rather than physical or situational. He is asking the professional to provide an explanation as to why he thinks, feels, or acts the way he does. The patient anticipates playing a passive role in the interaction, contributing only that information that the expert requires.

Psychodynamic insight. The patient perceives his problem as psychological in origin, as evolving from his early development, and as having a repetitive quality. As a result, he is left feeling unhappy, unfulfilled, but not overwhelmed or out of control. He expects to take an active, collaborative role in talking about the roots of his problem and hopes that a better understanding of his problem will enable him to change.

Reality contact. The patient feels that he is losing hold of reality. He wants to talk to someone who is psychologically stable and "safe." The request is for the clinician to help him "check out" or "keep in touch with" reality so that he will feel he is thinking straight and not losing his mind.

Social intervention. The patient sees the problem as residing primarily in the people or situations around him. Because he feels that he does not possess the resources to effect the necessary change, he is asking the clinic to intervene on his behalf. He is asking not for the legal powers of the clinic but for its social influence.

Succorance. The patient is feeling empty, alone, not cared for, deprived, or drained. He wants the clinician to care, to be involved, to be comforting, and to be warm and giving so that he can feel replenished and warm inside. It is not so much the content of the interchange that is requested as its affective quality of warmth and caring.

Ventilation. The patient would like to tell the clinician about various feelings and affect-laden experiences. The patient anticipates that "getting it out" or getting it off his chest will be therapeutic. He feels like he is carrying around a burden that he would like to leave with the clinician. In contrast to confession, the patient does not feel guilty and does not need or want forgiveness.

Nothing. Patients who make no request are a heterogeneous group. They may have been referred without proper preparation; they may be psychotic; they may have problems but are not seeking help at this time; they may want help but are reluctant to state the problem; they may not need help; they may be in the wrong clinic.

We have recently developed a 75-item questionnaire, the Patient Request Form (PRF), to measure requests in these 14 categories. Using this instrument, we have demonstrated by factor analytic techniques the mathematical independence of most of these request categories and have described the frequency with which patients make particular requests in a walk-in clinic.[4]

Since clinicians, after learning the patient's complaint (chief complaint) or the patient's goals, often believe they know the patient's request, it is worth distinguishing the three. The complaint is the patient's initial statement as to what is bothering him; for instance, "I am depressed." The goal is what the patient would like to accomplish or how he would like to feel; for instance, "I would like to feel well enough to return to work." It is the goal that is the basis of the "contract" of transactional analysis.[5] The request is how the patient would like the clinician to respond to help him achieve the desired goal. He might request *clarification:* "Help me understand the reasons why." He might request *social intervention:* "Tell my family to stop degrading me." He might request *medical* intervention: "Give me something for my nerves." He might make an *administrative* request: "Would you write a letter to my draft board?" In our studies of initial interviews, we have found that the complaint is invariably elicited, the goal is usually elicited, and the request is often *not* elicited. Clearly, the negotiation process will be seriously impaired if the clinician does not know the patient request.

Elicitation of the Patient Request

Since the patient's statement of the request during the initial interview is a critical beginning of the customer approach, how the clinician elicits the request deserves special attention.

Sometimes the patient will state the request spontaneously at the beginning of the interview. When this does not occur, the patient request is best elicited after learning the patient's complaint and a meaningful part of the present illness. This preliminary interaction establishes the rapport necessary for the elicitation of the patient request, which turns out to be a most intimate revelation. Eliciting the request at the very start of the interview before the patient has stated the problem increases the chances of placing the patient in the position of adversary rather than collaborator in the diagnostic and therapeutic process. "You asked me what I want. You do not even know what is wrong with me." Eliciting the request at the end of the interview deprives the clinician of the opportunity to negotiate or work with the request.

We have been most successful in eliciting the patient request by asking: "How do you hope (or wish) I (or the clinic) can help? The questions "What do you want?" or "What do you expect?"

should be avoided since they are apt to be perceived as a confrontation. The words "wish" or "hope," in contrast, give the patient permission to state requests he does not necessarily expect will be granted. Even when the clinician finally asks the patient what he hopes for, the response is commonly "I don't know. You are the therapist," or "I just want to feel better." In this kind of situation the patient frequently has a rather specific request in mind that he is reluctant to state for reasons we will describe later. The elicitation of the request then requires persistence, persuasion, and compassion. "You must have had some idea when you decided to come," or "It is important for me to know what your wishes are even if I may not be able to fulfill them."

The initial statement of the request may be incomplete or stated in such general terms that it requires elaboration to achieve the specificity necessary for clinical utility. "You said you want me to help you understand things better. What in particular do you want to understand?" or "You thought you would feel better if I would fix up your family situation. How do you hope I can fix it up?" When the request has finally been stated and elaborated, it is important that the clinician acknowledge that he/she has heard and understood the request. Otherwise, the patient may wonder whether the clinician heard the request, was offended by it, or didn't believe it worthy of a response.

The elicitation of the request undoubtedly depends on more than timing and phraseology. Certainly the clinician's attitude of interest and receptivity is crucial. We have observed, for instance, that the patient frequently hints at or alludes to the request apparently waiting for some response from the clinician that will indicate that it is acceptable to continue or to become more specific.

As the interview proceeds, the clinician should listen for elaborations of or changes in the request resulting from the developing relationship between clinician and patient. The patient thinks to himself, "Now that I have more trust in you, let me tell you what I really want," or "Now that you have responded to my initial request, it occurs to me that there is something more important that I need."

Negotiation and Disposition of the Patient Request

What we refer to as "negotiation" is the heart of the clinical process. It is the coming together, the interaction, the dialogue between the patient who is formulating what he thinks he needs and the clinician who is formulating what hopefully is clinically appropriate. In an ideal negotiation, the patient exerts his influence in several ways. First, since the request has considerable diagnostic value (see next section on "Clinical Implications"), the patient is providing the clinician with valuable information. Second, the statement of the request itself obliges the clinician to consider the legitimacy of the perceived need and to explain why an alternative formulation might be more valid. Third, the patient has the right to evaluate and ultimately accept or reject any treatment proposal. In the process he may expect to receive from the clinician a further explanation, an alternative treatment plan, or a statement that the staff cannot meet the request.

The clinician is simultaneously exerting influence by the clarification and evaluation of each request in regard to whether it is clinically appropriate, clinically sufficient, and clinically feasible. If a request is clinically inappropriate, such as a request for medications where there is little likelihood that medications will be effective or a request by a manic patient for psychoanalysis, the clinician attempts to educate the patient so that he will change his request.

It is not uncommon for the request to be appropriate, but not sufficient. For example, the patient who wants to talk out his upset feelings about his failing memory undoubtedly has a legitimate request, but he also may need a neurological referral. For the patient who on repeated occasions asks the clinic to intervene in repetitious social situations, the clinician might consider with the patient how he contributes to his own problem.

Where the request is clinically appropriate but not clinically feasible because of the limitations of the treatment facility, such as a scarcity of psychotherapy time or the absence of a laboratory to measure blood lithium levels, this dilemma should be stated directly and honestly to the patient. At least the patient has received clinical confirmation of what he needs and can be referred elsewhere.

Impasses in negotiations are common and remedial strategies are varied. It may be helpful to understand the patient's theory about the nature of his illness and to inquire what he has tried before. It may help to know the patient's fears about his "illness" and what he specifically does not want to happen. It may be helpful for the clinician to restate the formulation in the patient's terminology in order to facilitate communication. Where the clinical picture represents a discrete syndrome, such as some of the affective disorders, if the clinician describes the syndrome, its course, and treatment, this often influences the patient to accept what is needed. The clinician may influence a patient to accept a recommendation for psychotherapy by helping him understand the psychotherapeutic process. This may be facilitated by showing the patient how he unnecessarily contributes to his own suffering or by helping him experience some painful feelings associated with key psychological issues.

CLINICAL IMPLICATIONS

The following six cases, taken from the Acute Psychiatric Service of the Massachusetts General Hospital, are presented to further illustrate the customer approach and its clinical implications.

Case 1

A 40-year-old female, whose chart referred to her as a "chronic schizophrenic," was referred to the Psychiatry Clinic from the Medical Clinic where she stated her problem as "noise pollution." From her facial expression, her bizarre thought content, and the history of multiple state hospitalizations, it seemed highly probable that the diagnosis was correct. It was also noted that she had been to our clinic several times. Each time she was referred back to her local mental health center. Now, much to our embarrassment, she came to our Medical Clinic. The diagnosis, the history, and the manner of presentation made the clinician feel helpless and angry. He knew she was ill and that he was expected to help. He believed he had nothing to offer.

After 15 minutes of a rambling, circuitous interview, the clinician asked in frustration how she hoped he could help. She requested to be put "on a stronger pill." The patient was receiving chlordiazepoxide hydrochloride (Librium) but no antipsychotic medications. The clinician was immediately put at ease since the request was reasonable. He no longer felt helpless. The clinician was then able to explore how the patient's daughter, now 13 years of age, was beginning to talk too much and too loudly. This situation seemed to coincide with the onset of the delusion about noise pollution. In addition to a change in medication, the patient was willing to accept the recommendation for a supportive relationship to help her deal with the psychological demands of the adolescent daughter.

The patient concluded by explaining that she was no longer accepting our referrals to her local mental health center because they hospitalize her before listening to her, She had come to our Medical Clinic because she felt the Psychiatry Clinic, before today, had not listened to her either.

Case 2

A 27-year-old male presented with the target complaint of "nerves
. . . too much drinking." With considerable urgency he communicated
his goal of discontinuing drinking and specifically requested pills to accomplish the goal. The clinician, who felt the request was reasonable
but failed to share this belief with the patient, proceeded to inquire
into other areas that might help explain the drinking. Tension in the interview mounted. Finally the patient angrily responded, "My marriage
is okay, my family is okay, everything is okay . . . . Look, first give
me the pills and then I'll sing." With the request clearly stated, the
clinician assured the patient that he believed pills were indicated and
agreed to write a prescription at the end of the interview. The patient,
knowing that his request was heard and would be granted, proceeded
to describe his marital difficulties, which culminated in his striking his
wife. This loss of control was the final event that brought him to the
clinic.

Case 3

A 55-year-old hospital employee who presented to the clinic was interviewed by a psychiatric resident in the presence of three other residents
and the senior author. The patient said he was upset and depressed.
Some mild depressive symptomatology was indeed elicited. He further
explained that he was troubled by his wife's recent hospitalization
for a recurrent psychotic condition. The resident attempted to understand the depression in terms of his loneliness and/or his feelings of guilt
but was unable to elicit responses that would support this formulation.
The patient's request was not elicited.

The patient was asked to wait outside the office while the residents conferred about possible treatment options. Psychotherapy and
pharmacological treatments were considered. It was decided that the
request should first be elicited.

In response to the question "How did you wish we could help?"
the patient replied, "I work here in the hospital kitchen and bring
food up to the psychiatry ward. It's a nice clean place and they treat
the patients well. If you have space, would you call the state hospital
and have her transferred? I would feel much better."

The transfer was arranged and the patient became asymptomatic.

Case 4

A 42-year-old divorced female presented to the clinic with the following statement: "My house burned down 2 days ago. I need something
for myself; I need pills for my nerves." The patient was given the opportunity to tell her story for the next 30 minutes. She seemed to use
the time for ventilation, emotionally recounting in considerable detail
the description of the fire. The clinician's supportive listening was a

response to the first part of the patient's request for "something for myself." The clinician could then respond to the second part of the request with "I don't believe pills are necessary." The patient replied, "I agree with you. I'm feeling so much better already. Could you give me your name and phone number so I can call you and let you know how things work out?"

Case 5

An unkempt 46-year-old chronic alcoholic male, smelling of alcohol but not acutely intoxicated, was guarded during the first few minutes of the interview as he tried to sense whether he would receive the unfriendly welcome often given the alcoholic patient. As he began to feel that the clinician was interested in finding out what was bothering him and what he wanted, he proceeded to tell his story. Born in Scotland, he had only one relative in this country, a sister living in Baltimore. The patient had lost contact with her when she was hospitalized 8 months ago. He could never muster the nerve to call for fear of learning of her death. His request of the clinician was for *social intervention:* "Would you phone her for me? Here is 2 dollars and 30 cents." The clinician made the call and successfully put him back in contact with his only relative. (An implicit request was for the clinician to be with him if he learned of his sister's death.) The patient then told the clinician that his visit today was triggered by his bringing his only companion into the hospital for cirrhosis.

As the clinician heard the story, he considered and ruled out the possibility that the patient was suffering from impending delirium tremens, Wernicke's encephalopathy, or another condition that would have required some "negotiation" over necessary medical treatment.

Case 6

A 28-year-old single female came for help because of depression that was impairing her capacity to concentrate at work. The depression followed her rejection by a married man, 15 years her senior, whom she had felt close to for 5 years. She described this man in terms ("fascinating . . . never understood by his wife") similar to those she used to describe her father whose death she failed to grieve. It became apparent to the clinician that the depression was dynamically related to her unresolved feelings toward her father. The patient, who was bright and insightful, seemed to understand these issues. Near the end of the interview, the clinician elicited the patient request with full anticipation that she would want psychotherapy. Her response was "Give me pills to make me feel numb." The question immediately arose as to why the patient did not want psychotherapy. This led to a discussion of a traumatic termination of her previous psychotherapy. It was necessary to schedule a second interview to deal with the meaning of the prior termination before the patient would begin to work at her current dilemma.

Diagnostic Issues

The patient's response to the clinician's elicitation of the request provides information that is diagnostic in the broadest sense. Indeed, some diagnostic data may not become apparent—or will be delayed—unless the request is elicited. As a result of this information, the clinical process becomes more efficient and more effective.

There are many clinical situations in which the patient's statement of what he wants is exactly what he needs. Using the customer approach, the clinician has the chance to learn this information early in the interview and to profit from the patient's ideas, a commonly ignored source of diagnostic data. In Case 1, the patient with schizophrenia wanted and needed stronger medication. This information may have emerged later in the interview. However, in a busy clinical setting and with a history of frequent nonproductive visits, the patient may have been sent elsewhere before being adequately evaluated. In Case 2 the patient wanted and needed pills. In Case 3 the patient wanted and needed administrative assistance to obtain better care for his wife and to feel that he was doing all that was in his power to help her. If the request were not directly elicited, his needs would never have been known. In Case 4 the patient wanted and needed "something for myself." Had this part of the request not been made explicit, the clinician might have administered or withheld medicines without being aware of a more important need. In Case 5 the patient wanted and needed someone to put him in contact with his sister and to be available for other supportive needs if it were learned that his sister were dead. Unless the patient felt comfortable enough to make the request, he would have left with his needs unmet. The clinician may have commented, "Just another alcoholic."

When the patient's request is clinically appropriate, making a careful diagnosis of the request can be very important in determining the precise clinical response. Take, for example, the requests for *ventilation, confession,* and *reality contact* in three separate patients and assume that these requests represent valid clinical needs. An accurate diagnosis of the request/need will lead to three distinct clinical responses. For the patient who needs *ventilation,* the clinician can best help by taking the role of the interested listener. If the clinician breaks in to make interpretive comments, the patient is apt to tolerate the interruption, ignore the clinician's words, and go on with his story. For the patient who needs *confession*, the clinician can best help by an attitude and verbal response which puts the deed in a medical or psychological perspective (when the guilt is neurotic) or which (when guilt is real) shows compassion in helping the patient bear the painful feelings. If the clinician were to assume the role of the interested listener (as for *ventilation*), the patient would take this response as confirmation of his guilt. For the patient who needs *reality contact*, it may be important for the clinician to actively share thoughts about what is real. Again, the role of the passive listener might aggravate the condition.

The diagnostic value of the patient request is equally apparent when it seems out of the clinical context of the interview, clinically inappropriate, and/or when it catches the clinician unawares. If these situations arise, it is likely the clinician was on the wrong track in his interpretation of the complaint. This was the situation in Case 3 in which the hospital employee wanted the clinic to arrange for a transfer and in Case 6 in which the patient wanted medications to make her feel numb. The interview would have been more efficient and more effective in both these situations if the request had been learned earlier.

The patient's response to the clinician's elicitation of the request may also have special diagnostic meaning when the patient is reluctant to or refuses to state what he wants (see next section on "Resistance to the Customer Approach"). If the clinician pursues the matter, he will often learn important characterological information about the patient. Patients have told us, for instance, that they are not worthy enough to ask for anything, that they are unwilling to commit themselves, that they will be obligated to give the clinician something in return, etc. Without these responses, exploration of significant psychological issues may be delayed.

Process Issues

There is apt to be a great deal of wasted time and energy during an interview in which the patient request is verbalized either late in the interview or not at all. Instead of speaking freely about the problem, the patient may be preoccupied, wondering whether the clinician is kind enough, respectful enough, wise enough, understanding enough, and flexible enough to hear the request. "When will the clinician be ready to hear?" "When will I have the guts to come right out with it?" The clinician, meanwhile, often unaware of these concerns, goes about the business of establishing diagnoses and making treatment recommendations, not understanding why the patient participates only reluctantly during the interview. On the other hand, when the patient has stated the request early in the interview and feels it has been supportively heard, he is apt to participate more freely and feel more satisfied at the end.

Sometimes the clinician unwittingly discourages the patient from stating his request. One may observe in this situation a sparring between the clinician and the patient. For example, the patient throws out a hint about the request, "I think I may need to be watched over for a time (alluding to a request for hospitalization)." The clinician then changes the subject without acknowledging the request. "Have you had any physical illness recently?" He responds with hostility, "I'm just fed up with everything!"

Sometimes the patient, feeling there is no opening, waits until the end of the interview before stating the request: "By the way, would you . . . :" The clinician now has new and essential data but not enough time to evaluate or to act on it. For example, a patient comes to a medical clinic allegedly for a general exam. As he is about to leave the office after the examination, he states the real request: "Please tell me if I have cancer." Had the patient made the request earlier and had the clinician perceived the request as legitimate and important, the clinician could have explored the reasons for the patient's concern and learned what kind of explanation would be most appropriate.

In many clinical situations, acknowledging the request or giving the patient what he asks for satisfies needs that must be met before a healthier request can be made. For instance, patients who first request *control, reality contact,* or *succorance* cannot be expected to progress to requests requiring their active collaboration such as *clarification* until the more basic requests are dealt with. In Case 2 satisfying the request for medication frees the patient to explore social or psychotherapy requests regarding the marriage. We refer to this process of shifting requests from sicker to healthier as progressive. Contrariwise, patients whose initial requests are rejected or not acknowledged may subsequently present with a sicker or regressive request. For example, if a request for *social intervention* is denied, the patient may request *control* or *reality contact.* The chronic alcoholic patient, Case 5, may have had these needs had his request to phone his sister been denied.

The elicitation of the patient request has, in many situations, an important impact on the clinician that, in turn, affects the entire course of the interview. In Case 1, for instance, the clinician's feeling changed from anger to compassion upon learning that there was something to do. Similarly, the clinician in Case 3, before hearing the request for assistance in transferring his wife to the Massachusetts General Hospital, felt bewildered that neither medical nor psychodynamic formulations explained the patient's presentation. In Case 5, the "uncurable chronic alcoholic" became a human being in distress once his request became known.

It is not uncommon for overworked clinicians, often dealing with patient populations culturally different from their own, to believe that the patient wants radical changes in character and symptomatology that are hard to fulfill. The clinician further believes that the patient will expect these changes and then becomes angry at the patient for having such unreasonable demands. Having the patient state his request undercuts this series of projections since what the patient wants is almost always more modest than what the clinician had expected. Patients do not want to be different human beings. They want to feel better.

RESISTANCE TO THE CUSTOMER APPROACH

On the face of things, it would appear that the customer approach described above is no more than a psychological conceptualization of common sense or a statement of the obvious. It would seem hard to disagree with the idea that the clinician, after encouraging the patient to say what he wants, should gather more data and then educate and be educated by the patient so that in the end those requests that are clinically appropriate would be satisfied. We have, nevertheless, observed an extraordinary amount of resistance (not used in the psychoanalytic sense) on the part of clinicians and patients to this approach. It is as if there were a conspiracy between both parties in which the patient agrees not to say what he wants and the clinician agrees not to ask. This resistance is manifested in several ways:

1. In several clinics we have observed that in most initial interviews patients do not state their requests. Even when the clinician believes that the request has been elicited, our examination of the tape-recorded interview indicates this is often not the case. Furthermore, when the patient hints at or alludes to what he wants, the clinician commonly changes the subject, thereby indicating that the request is not important.

2. Given the seeming importance of knowing what patients request, there is a paucity of literature on the subject. The limited research on patient expectations addresses itself to what the patient anticipates will occur, not necessarily what he wants to occur. Beyond the statement that patients go for help, there is no elaboration of what help means to the patient.

3. When the customer approach is presented in the form described in this chapter, many audiences seem to misunderstand what has been said and become angry. The misunderstanding takes the form of hearing that clinicians should always do whatever the patient asks. Anger has been expressed in the form of "I don't care what the patient wants" or "What about the trainee's request; never mind the patient."

Resistance by the Clinician

Clinicians describe several reasons why they neither elicit nor respond to patient requests. Some believe that from hearing the target complaint and the goal, they know the patient's request even though it has not been made explicit. In other words, the clinician is apt to assume that a bright, intelligent, insightful person who describes some personality inadequacy wants psychotherapy. Other clinicians believe either that patients cannot verbalize what they want or that the verbalizations are conscious distortions of unconscious processes. For some, the issue of professional norms is at stake. It is feared that the patient will regard the clinician who elicits the patient's request as not professionally responsible. "You should know; you are the therapist." Another important issue has to do with authority. In these circumstances, the clinician may feel that asking the patient what he wants is tantamount to turning over the authority for treatment to the patient. But perhaps the most important issues that keep the clinician from finding out how the patient would like him to intervene are those of impotence and helplessness. There is the concern of many of us that eliciting the request will open up a Pandora's box of unending, overwhelming, and depleting demands that the clinician would rather avoid.

Resistance by the Patient

We have observed three major reasons why patients find it difficult to tell the clinician what they want. The first has to do with their perception that it is the patient's role to state his problem but not his evaluation of how the help should be provided. The patient, nevertheless, reserves the right to take his business elsewhere if he is not satisfied. The second reason has to do with the patient's perception of the clinic as the adversary who has the power to say no. As a result, the patient must hint at his request or present it in an indirect way that may maximize his chances of "winning." The third reason why patients find it difficult to say what they want has to do with a wide range of personality variables: (a) Some patients feel that making the request explicit diminishes the quality of the giving. "A caring clinician would know what I wanted without my asking." (This situation is similar to complimenting one's spouse's appearance only after he or she has requested it.) (b) Some patients may not feel worthy enough to ask, "Who am I to ask for anything?" (c) Others feel humiliation and loss of pride if they have to ask for anything. (d) Some patients feel that stating their wish leads to too much intimacy or closeness, that they could become too open or exposed and therefore subject to criticism, ridicule, rejection, or even acceptance and other feared positive feelings. (e) Patients may be concerned that saying what they want is limiting by making it unlikely that they will obtain more. By keeping the request vague, it is possible to receive more. (If you ask $30,000 for your house, no one will offer you $31,000.) (f) Others are reluctant to state what they want because they will have then committed themselves and are not psychologically prepared to do so, "If I say what I want, you may take me seriously and hold me to what I say." (g) Some patients fear that if they verbalize their desires, the magnitude of their needs might embarrass them. (h) Some patients fear that the clinician, by granting the request, would want something in return. (i) Some patients fear that if their request is granted, they would be forced to change their notion of the world as a mean, ungiving place. (j) Others fear that the clinician may yield to a request that may be clinically inappropriate. "He might do what I want and that might turn out to be a mistake." (k) Others may fear that the clinician, by saying yes to the request, will fail to set needed limits, "I needed him to say no!"

The difficulty in stating what one wants, wishes, or hopes for is hardly limited to the clinician–patient relationship. It is deeply rooted in our culture; for example, in making wishes after blowing out the candles or breaking the wishbone, children must keep the wish to themselves if it is to have the best chance of coming true. In seeking out certain academic and industrial positions, one does not ask for the job. The chances for attaining the position are enhanced if someone else submits the applicant's name.

COMMENT

Evidence is accumulating that psychiatric patients and the professionals who serve them are worlds apart.[7] This is especially true for patients of the lower social classes who constitute the major case load of many hospital clinics and community mental health centers. These patients frequently have goals and expectations of treatment that differ from the therapists who treat them.[7,8,9] Specifically, the patients of the lower classes want help with symptoms or unpleasant social conditions and they expect the professional to be active, warm, directive, medical in orientation, and willing to give advice. Clinicians, on the other hand, expect to be nondirective and "neutral," and they require their patients to be introspective and verbally active. The dropout rates of up to 60 percent after the first interview have been attributed to these discrepancies.[10,11] As a result of these findings, many clinicians and investigators have expressed doubts whether patients of the lower social classes could be treated by long-term psychotherapy.[13] These clinical practices emerged from an era in which long-term psychotherapy was virtually the only outpatient psychiatric treatment that had any respectability in this country and was considered by many to be the very essence of American psychiatry. Unfortunately, the applicant's need for treatment often became less important than his credentials for "suitability."

Two important developments in psychiatry are changing these practices. The first is the advances in technology (psychopharmacology, behavior therapy, family therapy, brief therapy, structural learning therapy,[13] etc.) that better enables the clinician to respond to a broad variety of patient complaints, requests, and needs. The second development is the financing and delivery of psychiatric services through community mental health centers and health maintenance organizations. These changes have resulted in greater accessibility to treatment for a broader range of patients, a commitment to treat all patients from a catchment area, a broader definition of psychiatric problems, and a new power relationship between patients and clinicians.

This change in the professional–client relationship, described by sociologists interested in health, is already upon us.[14,15,16] Indeed, it seems probable that the patient will increasingly view himself as a purchaser of services, a "well-paying customer in a buyer's market."[17]

Some professionals find the word *customer* crass. We believe it is a useful metaphor to describe a relationship in which the patient has the right to ask for what he wants, to negotiate, and to take his business elsewhere if he so desires, while the clinician has the obligation to listen, to negotiate, and to offer treatment that meets professional standards. This "customer" relationship, we believe, is in the interest of both parties. On the other hand, a relationship characterized either by the patient taking whatever he wants or can pay for (as in the supermarket) or by the clinician acting independently of the patient's wishes runs the risk of being ineffective or even destructive to both parties.

As mental health professionals enter into clinical situations arising from the technical advances and social changes described above, new clinical demands will be made of them. They will become frustrated and fatigued. We believe that this discomfort results not only from limitations in the diagnostic system and clinical formulations but from our approach to patients. In this chapter we have attempted to conceptualize for clinicians an approach to patienthood based on the mutual influence between clinician and patient. We believe this approach results in improved patient care, patient satisfaction, and staff morale.

REFERENCES

1. Lazare, A, Eisenberg, L: Psychiatric residency training: an outpatient first year program. *Seminars in Psychiatry 2*:201–210, 1970.
2. Lazare, A, Cohen, F, Jacobson, AM, Williams, MS, Mignone, RJ, Zisook, S: The walk-in patient as a 'customer': a key dimension in evaluation and treatment. *Amer. J. Orthopsychiat 42*:872–883, 1972.
3. Levinson, D, Merrified, J, Berg, K: Becoming a Patient. *Arch Gen Psychiatr. 17*:385–406, 1967.
4. Lazare, A, Eisenthal, S, Wasserman, L, Harford, TC: "The Customer Approach to Patienthood," *Arch. Gen Psychiat* (in press).
5. Holloway, WH, and Holloway, MM: "Change Now: An Introduction to Contractual Group Treatment with Transactional Analysis," Midwest Institute for Human Understanding, Akron, Ohio.
6. Hornstra, RK, Lubin, B, Lewis, RV, Willis, BS: Worlds apart: patients and professionals. *Arch Gen Psychiat 27*:553–557, 1972.
7. Overall, B, Aronson, H: Expectations of psychotherapy in patients of lower socio-economic class. *Am J Orthopsychiat 33*:421–430, 1963.
8. Heine, RW, Trosman, H: Initial expectations of the doctor-patient interaction as a factor in continuance in psychotherapy. *Psychiatry 23*:275–278, 1960.

9. Borghi, J: Premature termination of psychotherapy and patient-therapist expectations. *Amer J Psychother 22*:460–473, 1968.

10. Rosenthal, D, Frank, J: The fate of psychiatric clinic outpatients assigned to psychotherapy. *J Nerv Ment Dis 127*:330–343, 1958.

11. Coleman, JV, Dumas, R: Contributions of a nurse in an adult psychiatric clinic: an exploratory project. *Mental Hygiene 46*:448–453, 1962.

12. Hunt, RG: Social class and mental illness: some implications for clinical theory and practice. *Am J Psychiat 116*:1065–1069, 1960.

13. Goldstein, AP: *Structured Learning Therapy,* New York: Academic Press, 1973.

14. Reeder, LG: The patient-client as a consumer: some observations on the changing professional-client relationship. *J Health Soc Behav 13*:406–412, 1972.

15. Campbell, J: Working relationships between providers and consumers in a neighborhood health center. *Amer J Public Health 60*:97–103, 1971.

16. Hochbaum, GM: Consumer participation in health planning: toward conceptual clarification. *Amer J Public Health 59*:1698–1705, 1969.

17. Freidson, E: Profession of Medicine. New York, Dodd, Mead, 1970.

4
patterns of crisis

Crisis situations are critical points of focus in preventive mental health programs. Various health education groups who practice primary prevention have as their objective the teaching of strategies and alternatives for avoiding potentially stressful situations. Clinicians who intervene in a crisis may also practice secondary prevention by detecting early cases of emotional illness and by making effective referral to appropriate treatment agencies.

Community mental health staff are in daily contact with people who are in crisis. The patient who is hospitalized is in a situational crisis in that his normal life style is disrupted. A family member dealing with the news of the death of a loved one is in a crisis. The stress of hospitalization and of subsequent financial costs also can expose the individual to a crisis situation of an economic nature.

All clinicians should be knowledgeable in the concepts and principles specific to crisis work. This chapter and its companion, Chapter 5, will present an overview of issues within the field of crisis theory.

CONCEPTUAL FRAMEWORK

Over the past several years, social scientists and mental health clinicians have been studying the effects of crises on individuals, families, and communities. Crisis theory has begun to attempt systematically to define the differences between various types of crises. Crisis theorists and practitioners point to the difficulty in making precise distinctions, however, because of gaps in the current state of knowledge of the elements of crisis patterns such as stress, response, and settling the crisis. There are, however, certain concepts that are basic in understanding crisis behavior.

Homeodynamics: A Stable State

Many people live a good percentage of their life in some degree of homeostasis or balanced state. Although daily problems contain stressors that create stressful conditions, under usual circumstances, the person's emotional equilibrium returns to its previous level. Psychic equilibrium involves a balance between a person's personality structure, defenses, and adjustment mechanisms and the stress he experiences.

Humans may be viewed as part of a complex adaptive system that has a simple homeostatic or balanced system and the qualities of self-direction and self-organization unique to high-level adaptive systems. The steady and unsteady state of human adaptive systems have been described by Ruth Wu as follows.[1]

> *Homeostasis:* describes a physiological balance, and homeostatic disequilibrium describes a physiological imbalance.
>
> *Stability:* describes a behavioral balance, and instability describes a behavioral imbalance.
>
> *Steady state:* describes the equilibria of both forces, physiological and behavioral; and an upset in the steady state is termed a system imbalance.

Health organization, therefore, requires the presence of both physiological homeostasis and behavioral stability. A diagram of these relationships is shown on page 57. It is important to remember that behavioral stability may occur in the absence of

[1] Ruth Wu, *Behavior and Illness* (Englewood Cliffs, N.J.: Prentice-Hall, Inc., 1973), p. 90.

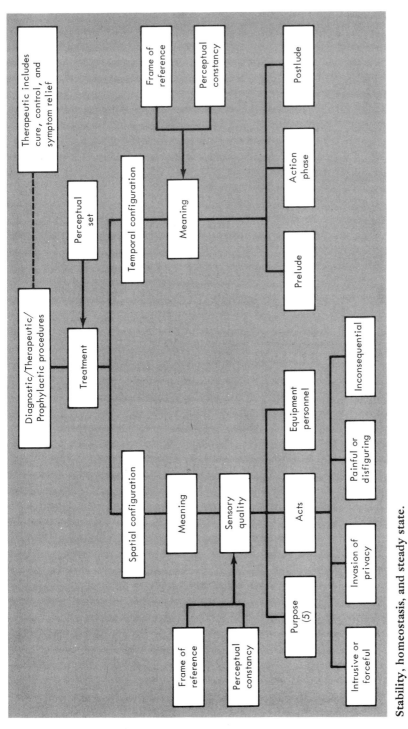

Stability, homeostasis, and steady state.
Ruth Wu, BEHAVIOR AND ILLNESS© 1973, p. 91. Reprinted by permission of Prentice-Hall, Inc., Englewood Cliffs, New Jersey.

homeostasis and conversely, if not prolonged, homeostasis may occur in the absence of behavioral stability. However, the absence of either one destroys the steady state.[2]

Stress

Research is underway by aviation safety human factors analysts on the relationship of stress factors to accident behavior. Dr. Robert A. Alkov emphasizes that the majority of accident behavior "can be explained by personal stresses which cause a person to perform in such a manner as to increase his or her accident liability."[3] These stresses are often transitory in nature and may be produced internally or originate from the external world.

In a study by Richard Rahe and Thomas Holmes,[4] 394 persons were asked to rate the amount of social readjustment required for each of the 43 life events listed most frequently by patients. The LCU (life change units) and calculated weights are shown in Table 4-1.[5]

Various studies are in progress comparing the relationship of a person's number of LCUs and his health status. In one pilot study of persons who had LCUs over 300 units, 79 percent had injuries or illness to report. In the studies, no particular event is linked to a particular disease. Undesirable events—the death of a spouse, for example—might produce severe depression. Preliminary findings are that a total of life events, each not in itself expecially undesirable, frequently leads to infection, allergy, or accidental injury, and the total impact of life events that require coping behavior predispose the person to a lowered ability to cope with illness or subsequent stress.[6]

The fact that people under stress may be more prone to illness and accident is not new. The development of scales to measure life change crises may be a useful assessment guide for the clinician—to monitor how much stress is in his client's, his staff's, or his own life. Such stress can affect one's performance and the kind of coping strategy that is available to him.

[2] Ibid.

[3] Robert A. Alkov, "Life Changes and Accident Behavior," *Approach: A Naval Safety Center Publication* (February 1975), pp. 18–20.

[4] Richard H. Rahe, "Life Crisis and Health Changes," Report No. 67-4, Navy Medical Neuropsychiatric Research Unit, San Diego, Calif.

[5] Adapted from Robert A. Alkov, "Life Changes and Accident Behavior," p. 19.

[6] Ibid., p. 20.

TABLE 4-1. Life Change Units

family constellation	mean value
Death of spouse	100
Divorce	73
Separation	65
Death of close family member	63
Marriage	50
Marital reconciliation	45
Change in family member's health	44
Pregnancy	40
Gain new member to family	39
Sexual difficulties	39
Arguments with spouse	35
Children leaving home	29
Trouble with in-laws	29
Change in living conditions	25
Move or change in residence	20
Change in schools, recreation, church activities, and social activities	20 19
Change in sleeping habits	16
Change in number of family get-togethers	15
Change in eating habits	15
Vacation	13
Holidays	12

individual changes	
Jail term	63
Personal injury or illness	53
Death of a close friend	37
Outstanding personal achievement	28
Revision of personal habits	24
Minor violation of the law	11

employment and/or school	
Fired at work	47
Retirement	45
Business readjustment	39
Change in job	36
Change in work responsibility (promotion or demotion)	29
Spouse begins or stops work	26
Begin or end school	26
Trouble with boss	23

financial	
Change in financial status	38
Mortgage or loan over $10,000	31
Foreclosure	30
Mortgage or loan under $10,000	17

Coping Mechanisms

When faced with a stressful situation, a person attempts to problem-solve through a mechanism called coping. These problem-solving efforts, according to Lazarus, Averill, and Opton, are made "by an individual when the demands he faces are highly relevant to his welfare (that is, a situation of considerable jeopardy or promise), and when these demands tax his adaptive resources."[7] This definition (1) emphasizes the importance of the emotional context in coping, (2) includes the stress component of emotion as well as the potential fulfillment or gratification element, (3) recognizes the overlap between problem-solving and coping, and (4) emphasizes adaptive tasks that are neither automatic nor routine.[8]

Coping strategies are immediate efforts employed by a person in attempting to meet and overcome the demands inherent in the stressful situation. Reactions to stress are attempts by an individual to defend himself against disorganization or an unstable state of physical and emotional health.

Crisis

When a person is faced with a change in his life situation in which there is a problem he cannot solve through his usual coping strategies, his emotional equilibrium is disrupted. If his homeostatic balance is unsuccessful in maintaining balance within a short period of time (from hours to a few days), the protracted period of disruption in life style is termed a crisis. According to Dr. Gerald Caplan, a crisis is associated with (1) a rise in inner tensions; (2) signs of unpleasant emotional feeling; and (3) disorganization of functioning.[9]

One's emotional state cannot remain in this crisis position indefinitely. One observes the signs of the acute emotional upset subside and some kind of adaptation or reorganization occurs. A new level of emotional equilibrium is reached. The person may be

[7] Richard S. Lazarus, James R. Averill, and Edward M. Opton, Jr., "The Psychology of Coping: Issues of Research and Assessment," *Coping and Adaptation.* Edited by George V. Coelho, David A. Hamburg, and John E. Adams (New York: Basic Books, Inc., 1974), pp. 250–251.

[8] Ibid.

[9] Gerald Caplan, *Concepts of Mental Health and Consultation* (Washington, D.C.: U.S. Government Printing Office, 1959), p. 185.

as stable or mentally healthy as he was previous to the crisis; the person may be less emotionally stable, or the person may have gained in emotional strength. Thus, crisis is a time in one's life when one can either gain strength psychologically or regress to a mental ill-health level.

TYPOLOGY OF CRISES

Clinicians talk of two main types of crisis: the internal or maturational crisis of the life cycle, and the external or situational crisis.

Internal Crises

Sigmund Freud's theory of psychosexual development and Erik Erikson's formulation of the eight stages of development in the human life cycle provide the theoretical basis for analyzing developmental or maturational crises. Erikson conceptualizes personality development as a succession of differentiated phases, such as infancy, childhood, adolescence, and adulthood, each being qualitatively different from its predecessor. Between one phase and the next, periods of transition are characterized by disorganized behavior. The person may be aware of minor mood swings as well as fluctuating emotions and thoughts experienced during the phase. The solution arrived at from the previous phase is then applied to the next phase. Erikson emphasizes the relationship between the person's social development and his social environment. He also emphasizes the normal aspect of the stages of development. For example, he goes into considerable detail in describing the normal "identity crises" in the adolescent developmental crisis phase, stating that the phase includes increased conflicts with which the person must deal concurrently.

Erikson identifies these eight major developmental crises in terms of the tasks that must be resolved in each phase. They are in chronological order: basic trust versus mistrust; autonomy versus shame and doubt; initiative versus guilt; industry versus inferiority; identify versus role confusion; intimacy versus isolation; generativity versus stagnation; and ego integrity versus despair.

Internal or developmental crises are expected events occurring normally to most individuals in the course of their life span. Because they are expected, an individual has the opportunity during his development to prepare for these events. This approach is designed and encouraged by clinicians to decrease the crisis experience and increase the person's internal control over the normal event.

Mastery of these internal crises play a large part in determining the ego strength of the individual. Coping skills are tried and tested to deal with the various maturational tasks.

For example, considerable interest and study is being exerted in the area of sex role stereotyping and how men and women are coping with the division of labor when they have a two-career family.[10] The tasks involved in the two-career family very often include entertaining, housekeeping, and child care. In a study by a sociologist, Dr. Lynda Lytle Holmstrom, various coping strategies were identified by couples willing to try other than traditional methods of coping with tasks. For example, couples reported increasing the efficiency of housework through the use of machines or streamlining or eliminating certain housework tasks. Some couples described lowering standards for housekeeping. They were able to tolerate and accept untidiness in their homes in substitution for having two careers. Other couples paid for additional housekeeping services such as having a housekeeper to do the work they did not have time for. The task of child rearing was mastered through increased husband participation in parenting, modified work schedules, and hired help.[11] Coping strategies, thus, play a key role in the ability of a man and woman to each pursue a meaningful career without sacrificing the maturational tasks of intimacy and parenting.

The negative settlement of a maturational crisis may be termed a "fixation" and often leads to a characterological defect. Such difficulties interfere with the person's interpersonal relationships, and correcting of the defect may require psychotherapy.

Research projects are studying such maturational crises. One multidisciplinary research project dealt with the issue of further understanding the coping tasks and significant emotional and psychological adjustments of a mother's new role as a parent. The mother who is unable to cope with this developmental task of mothering may suffer a maturational crisis termed puerperal breakdown.[12]

---

[10] Lynda Lytle Holmstrom, *Two-Career Family* (Cambridge, Mass.: Schenkman, 1972).

[11] Ibid., p. 59–83.

[12] Henry Grunebaum, Justin L. Weiss, Bertram J. Cohler, Carol R. Hartman, and David H. Gallant, *Mentally Ill Mothers and Their Children* (Chicago: The University of Chicago Press, 1975).

Dr. Carol Hartman, a psychiatric clinician, describes the acute disequilibrium as being expressed in the mother's attitudes toward,
and treatment of, her family. The new mother-infant relationship
is particularly vulnerable to the mother's sense of failure and dissatisfaction in other aspects of her life. Signs and symptoms of the
mother's breakdown are: emotional detachment, withdrawal, intense involvement marked by inconsistency and impulsiveness,
poor judgment in assessing the baby's needs, and seemingly irreconcilable conscious or unconscious negative feelings toward the
baby. Dr. Hartman states, "Underscoring these reactions is her
conscious awareness of extreme and inexplicable displeasure in
caring for her baby; she senses her failure."[13]

External Crises

Anticipated life events. Anticipated life events may be non-
traumatic, growth-promoting, or hazardous. In a study by Dr. J.
Steven Heisel and his associates [14] specific life events were identified in the life cycle of the child, adolescent, and young adult.
These life events are important to understand because all events
involve stress which implies a need for coping as well as possible
adaptive measures if the event is seen as hazardous. These anticipated life events may be identified as follows and always involve
a certain degree of participation by the person. That is, the situation is usually agreed upon by the person; the hazardous event
may be superimposed.

School related: beginning nursery school, first grade, seventh grade, or
high school; change to a different school; failure of a year in school;
being accepted into a college of one's choice.

Family-related: birth or adoption of a brother or sister; change of
father's occupation requiring increased absence from the home; marital
separation of a parent; divorce of a parent; marriage of a parent to a
step-parent; addition of a third adult to the family (e.g., grandparent,
aunt, uncle); change in parents' financial status; increase or decrease in
number of arguments between parents as well as with parents.

Self-related: having a visible congenital deformity; change in acceptance by peers; outstanding personal achievement; becoming involved

---

[13] Ibid., p. 85–86.
[14] J. Steven Heisel, Scott Ream, Raymond Raitz, Michael Rappaport,
and R. D. Coddington, "The Significance of Life Events as Contributing Factors
in the Diseases of Children, III: A Study of Pediatric Patients," *Journal of Pediatrics* 83, No. 1 (1973), 119–123.

with drugs or alcohol; failing to be involved in an extracurricular activity one wished to join such as band or athletic team; breaking up with boyfriend or girlfriend; beginning to date; fathering an unwanted pregnancy; unwed pregnancy.

Unanticipated life events. A crisis may occur when an unexpected traumatic external event is effective in disrupting the balance between a person's internal ego adaptation or homeostatic state and the environment. The crisis is an interaction between an extreme external stressor and the adaptive capacity of the person. The unexpected nature of the event and the coping resources of the person will determine the dimensions of the crisis experience.

These unexpected life events are usually chance events and unpredictable from the point of view of the person affected. It is the element of unpreparedness that triggers the crisis potential and reduces the person's control or mastery in the situation.

These hazardous events may be related to a failure such as in school, in work, or with an individual person; a death of an important person; imprisonment of a family member or friend; hospitalization of a family member or oneself.

Research studies are looking at such events as the birth of a handicapped child, the birth of a premature infant, and widowhood. These problems often demand solutions that are new for the individual who has never had to face up to such a scene. These situations are specific events that the person has to cope with in addition to the developmental task being faced.

Dr. Erik Lindemann's classical work on grief[15] has provided the main focus for understanding the symptomotology of the bereavement crisis. From his experience with bereaved individuals, Lindemann continued his research around the concept of emotional crisis. He identified certain inevitable events in human life that were potentially hazardous. Each situation contains emotional strain in which stress would be expanded and would necessarily call for additional resources or adaptive behavior. Such behavior in turn would lead to either mastery or failure.

Victim crises. There are life situations in which an individual faces an overwhelmingly hazardous situation and in which the individual may be physically or psychologically injured, traumatized, destroyed, or sacrificed. Such an event involves a physically

---

[15] Erik Lindemann, "Symptomatology and Management of Acute Grief," *American Journal of Psychiatry* **101**, No. 1 (1944), 141–148.

aggressive and forced act identified by another person, a group of persons, or by an environment.

Examples of such victim crises are national disasters such as war, civilian disasters such as riots and racial persecutions, and violent crimes such as murder, rape, and assaults.

Not only crisis theorists but other disciplines are taking an increased interest in the victim. For example, people interested in law and criminology have also begun to look at the victim. B. Mendelsohn, an attorney, takes credit for proposing the term "victimology"—the study of the victim—in order to develop an independent field of investigation. And a major study was made regarding the criminal and his victim by Hans von Hentig. Over a 25-year period, the number of publications relevant to study and understanding the victim in various situations has increased considerably.[16]

In studying victim description of the crisis experience, four phases which vary in intensity and duration were noted.[17] The first phase is an early awareness of danger. Not all victims will or can describe this phase. It involves a psychological process that intervenes between the stress event and one's coping behavior or the appraisal of the degree of danger, threat, or harm.[18] Very often this phase is described as a "sixth sense" or a feeling of impending danger.

The second phase is the threat of attack and this is the point when the person realizes there is a definite danger to his life. The coping task at this stage is to try and avoid the danger.

The third phase in a victim experience is coping with the actual danger such as being robbed or physically assaulted. The coping task at this stage is to survive the danger despite whatever demands are made on the victim.

The last phase—after the victim experience and the coping task—is to be free or escape from the assailant or the situation. Various coping strategies are again used in this stage.

Speculating whether or not a crisis will develop after a victim experience is an important clinical concern. The question is not whether a crisis will develop, but rather the ripple effect or

[16] Ann Wolbert Burgess and Lynda Lytle Holmstrom, *Rape: Victims of Crisis* (Bowie, Md.: Robert J. Brady Company, 1974).

[17] Ann Wolbert Burgess and Lynda Lytle Holmstrom, "Coping Behavior of the Rape Victim" (Paper presented at the Annual American Psychiatric Association Meeting, Anaheim, Calif., May 8, 1975).

[18] Lazarus, Averill, and Opton, "The Psychology of Coping: Issues of Research and Assessment," p. 260.

the severity of disruption and disorganization during the acute phase of the crisis and the length of time for the reorganization back to a normal life cycle.

We believe that all life events are stressors and have the capacity to disrupt the homeostatic status of one's life style. The life event has the potential to disrupt multiple areas of a life style, and it is these areas which have a cumulative or ripple effect.

For example, a 32-year-old woman had moved into an urban city after ending a marriage of 3 years as well as a job of 10 years. She had recently moved into a new area and apartment and was seriously injured when she was assaulted and robbed. The subsequent hospitalization was a disruption to her life physically and emotionally. The situation also involved financial aspects which created a personal and financial crisis. Her physical recovery will be one part of her return to her normal life style. She has additional areas of her life to put back into order and all at a time when she is settling her feelings about dissolving a marriage, a job, and moving to a new environment.

ASSESSMENT

The initial interview of a crisis situation is a prime therapeutic entry point. The person is often under considerable tension and stress and will be very sensitive to the attitude and reaction of the clinician. The interview provides the clinician with the opportunity to observe the client, assess the crisis and the amount of stress the person is experiencing as well as to determine the model of care most useful to the person in the days and weeks to follow.

Establishing an Alliance

The purpose of establishing an alliance as quickly as possible is to help the client understand that the meeting between him and clinician is designed to help. In order for the client to trust the clinician and to be able to fully recount the details of the crisis, he has to see that there is something in the meeting for him. Without some degree of trust, the client may be reluctant to talk. This point is especially important in working with children and adolescents in crisis.

The clinician can encourage trust by treating the client with respect, helping to bear some of the distress that the client is experiencing, being honest, trustworthy, and empathetic. The ability of the clinician to have a calming effect on the client will be the key to reducing the client's tension and anxiety to more bearable limits.

Identifying the Crisis

By paying close attention to the first phrases of the clinical encounter, the crisis may well be identified. Sometimes it will be stated in the presenting complaint. Other times, the crisis will be more implicit and the clinician will have to listen carefully for the crisis issue.

Once the crisis has been identified, the clinician should try to keep the content focused on details of the crisis. The goal in crisis intervention is to understand as much of the incident as possible and the reactions of the person.

The clinician would want to know the circumstances under which the event occurred, the people involved, the conversation, the thoughts and reactions displayed by people, and significant events since the incident.

Perception of the Crisis Event

It is important to understand how the person views the crisis. The crisis the person faces can also be analyzed by looking at the interaction between his current developmental phase and the externally imposed event. The crisis takes on specific meaning to the person according to his stage of development in the life cycle. For example, psychiatrists Malkah Notman and Carol Nadelson state that the middle-aged woman who is raped is in a period of critical reassessment of her role, particularly in the face of menopausal concerns and her usefulness in relation to her now-absent family. Husbands in their own midlife crises are often less responsive and supportive to this victim crisis. Thus, the overwhelming life-threatening experience and autonomy-shaking rape is particularly damaging. It is a misconception that a woman past her earlier sexually most active period has less to lose than a younger woman when she is raped. Actually the opposite is true. The self-devaluation, feelings of worthlessness, dirtiness, and shame can be particularly acute in a female already sensitive to her sexual adequacy.[19]

[19] Malkah T. Notman and Carol C. Nadelson, "The Rape Victim: Psychodynamic Considerations" (Paper presented at the Annual American Psychiatric Association Meeting, Anaheim, Calif., May 8, 1975.)

The clinician can assess if the person is able to view the positive and negative factors of a crisis: are they evenly balanced or are they balanced too heavily on the negative side? To what degree will this alter the life style of the person?

Social Matrix Support

The clinician needs to assess who are the important people to the client. Does the client plan to tell or not tell them of the crisis? How have people responded to the client in previous difficulties? How secure is the person in his social network? The task is to put the person in touch with supportive and sensitive people; therefore, this type of assessment data is crucial.

Personality Structure and Coping Style

Studies have shown that people cope in a multitude of ways to stress and crisis situations.[20] Some people use cognitive strategies, such as thinking and planning what to do. Others use physical action or verbal strategies. Defense or mental mechanisms are psychological strategies that a person may use consciously or unconsciously.

The clinician can inquire as to what coping style the person has previously used and whether it has been effective and useful to the person. The clinician can also help distinguish what might be different about this crisis from other crises the person has encountered.

Eliciting the Crisis Request

The importance of finding out what the client wants in terms of professional services has been emphasized in Chapter 3. People in crisis may have additional requests, such as needing police or legal intervention. Therefore, the clinician should elicit the crisis request and attempt to negotiate clinical services to meet the request.

Diagnosis: Case Formulation

The clinician gathers all available data relevant to the crisis situation. This is data gathered from the individual, the social network, other additional sources such as previous contact with professionals and agencies.

[20] Burgess and Holmstrom, "Coping Behavior of the Rape Victim."

Crisis formulation includes a description of the precipitating events leading to the crisis, the perception of the stressful situation by the individual and the social network, the support the individual has available, and the individual's strengths and weaknesses with specific focus on coping skills. The type of crisis needs to be defined as to whether it is an anticipated life event, an unanticipated life event, or a victim experience.

INTERVENTION

The crisis state, as viewed by the helping person or agency, may be viewed as a therapeutic opportunity for the following reasons: the person, because his coping skills are not adequate, is now ready to learn new coping skills. He also may be in a better position to restrengthen ties with his social network with which he may previously have been alienated. For example, the teenager who withdrew from parents for various reasons may be now inclined to talk with parents because of the crisis situation. If the teenager is on drugs and has become overinvolved with their use, it may be possible to resolve the issue if the parents become involved as helping people.

The goal of crisis intervention is to offer help to the person in crisis so that the psychological equilibrium can be restored. The clinician tries to utilize all possible social network people who are important to the individual. The intervention should be as brief as possible and should focus on the immediate problem the person is facing. Some interventions may consist of one or two sessions. As soon as other significant (to the individual) people can be brought into the situation and these ties cemented, the crisis intervenor may assume a less active role and soon leave the situation.

Intervention Models

Problem-solving partnership. Barrell discusses the problem-solving partnership model as one type of intervention technique.[21] This approach emphasizes: (1) active involvement and participation by the intervenor and client in crisis therapy; (2) focusing and authenticating the crisis; (3) assessment; (4) generating an intervention plan; (5) implementation; (6) anticipatory planning, summary, and evaluation.

[21] Lorna Mill Barrell, "Crisis Intervention: Partnership in Problem-Solving," *Nursing Clinics of North America* 9, No. 1 (1974), 5–17.

Crisis counseling. This model of crisis intervention may be contrasted to the traditional psychotherapy model. Crisis counseling is issue-oriented and behavior difficulties of the past are not explored and are actively discouraged in the interview. In the initial interview material is obtained relevant to the crisis and the events leading to it. The assessment issues are explored. The interview is directive and structured. The crisis issue is subsequently defined in the client's terms and the degree of disruption to life style is evaluated together with the client. The goal of counseling is agreed to by the client and clinician. The plan for intervention is made and may continue with office visits or other techniques.[22]

Telephone counseling. The telephone, used as a crisis technique, is gaining acceptance as an intervention model. Suicide crisis centers have relied on the telephone to help talk people out of a suicidal act and Alcoholics Anonymous uses the telephone to provide its members access to another human being in hopes of everting a drinking episode. The telephone is also used widely in pediatrics so that the parent can call and talk with the pediatrician or pediatric nurse practitioner about a problem with the child. Health care centers are using the telephone routinely to do follow-up on patients.

The telephone is especially useful in crisis work for several reasons.

1. It provides relatively quick access to the person one wishes to contact.
2. The burden is not placed on the person in crisis to seek out help, make the appointment to see the crisis worker, and travel to an office at her own time and expense—all when she is in a crisis state and having difficulty making any decisions. Instead, the crisis worker initiates the intervention, seeks out the client and offers the service.
3. The client has considerable power in the situation and can say if she wishes to talk or not.
4. The client is able to resume a pre-crisis life style as quickly as possible. She does not have to further disrupt her life by adding office visits. It also reinforces the view that the person is considered "normal" rather than "sick" and in need of therapy. The client does not

[22] Donna C. Aguilera, Janice M. Messick, and Marlene S. Farrell, *Crisis Intervention: Theory and Methodology.* Second Edition (St. Louis: CV Mosby Company, 1974).

have to assume the sick role which therapy and the label of patient do connote to many people.

5. It is cost effective. It uses fewer resources—time, energy, and money—than do many other intervention methods.

The clinician uses telephone counseling to assess the progress of the client noting especially the symptom picture over time; that is, both physical and emotional symptoms and any other area of disruption to the person's life style. The nurse can identify the crisis and counseling request and respond to the request appropriately.[23]

Home counseling. Home visits are an additional method of crisis intervention and can be used when telephone counseling does not suffice. Other reasons for using home counseling are to reach a client without a telephone, to reach a client uncomfortable with the telephone and office visit, especially a child or family in crisis; to introduce oneself face-to-face as a member of a crisis intervention team; to obtain additional information by direct observation; and to facilitate group discussion within a family or social network. This added aspect of visual observation is the key difference in this method as contrasted with telephone counseling or with even an office visit if dimensions of the social network are important to understand.

Case Illustration

A 28-year-old mother of three children called the crisis unit of a community mental health center. In a very distressed tone of voice, she stated that her 5-year-old son had a "bad temper" and she could not control him. She described wanting to "hit and beat him" but was feeling guilty about having such feelings and needed help.

She related that one week previous her son was playing with a neighbor boy and wanted a toy the child had. He pushed the child and he subsequently fell and hit his head. The boy's mother was very upset and told the client that she should discipline her son more and that there was "something wrong with him to do such a thing."

The nurse at the crisis unit listened to the client and in a 10-minute conversation did an assessment of the mother in a situational crisis involving disciplining her five year old son. Her normal coping skills were not available and she felt she would "lose control and beat the

[23] Burgess and Holmstrom, *Rape: Victims of Crisis*, pp. 163–177.

child." The nurse asked if she might make a home visit to talk further about the situation and also to see the child. Together they could talk about the problem.

The nurse was not aware of the precipitating events and did not know the mother well enough to be able to identify her coping skills; however, the mother expressed her concern of losing control in the situation. The nurse made a visit to the home the next day and the following data was obtained.

The mother was verbal and easily discussed her feelings of frustration in dealing with her children all day long. Once during the conversation the 5-year-old son and 4-year-old sister started fighting over who was going to sit in the chair closest to the mother. The nurse observed the mother becoming more tense as evidenced by her chain smoking and talking faster and louder. Her attempts to set verbal limits on the children were abortive. The nurse intervened and asked the son to sit on the couch with her. This developed some dialogue with the child and the sister quietly sat in the chair. After a few moments the children decided to go outside to play.

The dialogue continued with the mother saying that she was upset over her fear of losing control and beating her children. The nurse pursued this association, and the mother soon revealed the fact that as a child she had witnessed her father murder her mother by physical assault. The mother was fearful that she was like her father and she sees her son in herself.

The nurse commented on this information by saying, "You are indeed concerned about your angry feelings and are fearful of them. It might be helpful to see how you can deal with these feelings when you are upset with your children so that you are not afraid of them."

This line of discussion led to talking about setting limits on the children's behavior, and the example of the fighting over the chair was used. The nurse helped the mother to see that talking about the fighting was an alternative to direction action of fighting. Other basic principles of setting limits on children's behavior was discussed such as how to intervene verbally as well as physically. Holding a child, as the nurse offered to the son during the chair fight, was discussed more in detail.

The nurse and mother agreed on the crisis issue: setting limits on the children's behavior. The stresser was the incident the week before when the neighbor-mother suggested that something might be wrong with the son. This remark stirred up old conflicting feelings about how anger and aggressive feelings are handled within the family. Talking about this as the stressful event decreased the mother's anxiety and helped her to see that her son was not her father and that she also was not her father.

The nurse said she could help the mother with the technique of parenting—that certain phases were more stressful than others. The nurse identified this as a crisis situation but also acknowledged that the incident involving the father and mother of this woman was an unresolved issue and that she might think of getting some help to talk that out sometime. The mother agreed but said she was more concerned with her day-to-day dealings with her children. The nurse suggested a mothers' group that was run by the visiting nurse association where issues of parenting were discussed. The mother agreed to this because she also wanted to talk with other women. The social aspects of this treatment method were most necessary because the mother felt isolated within the confines of her home.

A 6-month follow-up of the crisis situation indicated that the mother was faithfully attending the mothers' group which helped her feelings of isolation. Her fears of losing control with her children had been faced and was moving on to discuss other issues within the group.

Hospitalization. The use of hospitalization as an intervention method to crisis work has been documented primarily in crisis situations involving physical trauma and psychological disequilibrium. Also failure to deal with the maturational tasks of motherhood may bring a woman to the hospital. An intervention designed to aid mother and child in coping with the maturational task is a joint admission.[24] Such a situation helps the mother to experience her difficulties in mothering in an environment where problems can be dealt with as they arise. Focusing attention on the maturational crisis aids in preventing further withdrawal from mothering and lowered self-confidence.[25]

Evaluation

The best method to evaluate the effectiveness of crisis intervention is to match the verbal and behavioral response of the client in terms of the stated objective or goal. In the cited example, the mother felt that she had returned to her precrisis state. Her behavior was consistent with the self respect. She had not lost con-

---

[24] Grunebaum *et al.*, *Mentally Ill Mothers and Their Children.*
[25] Ibid.

trol of her anger. Rather, she was able to set realistic verbal and physical limits on all her children.

The client, if the intervention is successful, is back to a precrisis life style. The client reviews her precrisis life style, identifies the disruption caused by the crisis, and evaluates the current life style.

SUMMARY

This chapter discusses the research and clinical development in the field of crisis theory. A typology of crises is presented to include developmental crises that are the internal tasks that must be mastered as one progresses through the life cycle; external crises that are situational events that may be anticipated, unanticipated, or victim experiences in origin. Assessment, intervention, and evaluation of crises in the process complete the chapter.

5

issues in mental health consultation

Consultation has become an increasingly important skill in community mental health practice. This technique was originally developed and described by Dr. Gerald Caplan from his work in Israel and later at Harvard University. Mental health consultation has a close alliance with crisis work. The presence of a crisis situation provides certain advantageous factors for the clinician in helping a client. This chapter discusses mental health consultation in crisis and noncrisis situations, the process of consultation, and implications for consultant and consultee.

REQUESTS FOR CONSULTATION

Consultation involves two professionals (consultant and consultee) and the consultee's client, who usually has a mental health problem. The consultee requests the consultant's help on a difficult problem that he believes is within the consultant's specialized field. The consultant tries to obtain a maximum effect in a minimum amount of time.[1] There are many situations that may benefit from the use of consultation. They are discussed on the following pages.

Individual Request

A common consultation request will be the identification of a specific problem, for example, a patient whose behavior is creating stress to the overall functioning of a hospital ward. The mental health consultant within a hospital setting is often called on in this situation, which exemplifies consultation in a crisis situation. Depending on the consultation contract, the consultant works with the patient individually or works with the staff members who in turn will deal with the problem with the patient. The following illustrates one such situation:

> A mental health nursing consultant was called to a psychiatric inpatient unit of a general hospital and presented with the following problem by the head nurse: A 16-year-old female patient had been admitted on a Friday night. Over the weekend her behavior became exceedingly disruptive to the ward milieu. All methods to set limits on her behavior failed, and the physician made the decision to discharge her 4 days after admission. The patient began to complain that this action was unfair and said, "Staff should help the patient and not just throw her out." Staff discussed the issue and decided a staff–patient meeting should be held in order to help patients with their feelings about the situation. The decision had been made, but the patients made it clear at the combined meeting that they wished the decision reversed. After the meeting, the staff discussed their own ambivalent feelings and questioned what to do next since the patients were very upset over the decision.

The nursing consultant was asked for her opinion on the situation. This was a direct consultation request made by the head nurse to the consultant, and the dialogue continued between the two. The consultant gave her suggestions and the head nurse then had the additional input that provided more alternatives from which to make a decision.

[1] Gerald Caplan, *Concepts of Mental Health and Consultation* (Washington, D.C.: U.S. Government Printing Office, 1959), p. 149.

Group Identification of Problem

Often the consultation contract will be made between the consultant and a group such as an agency or the nursing staff of a unit within the hospital. The consultation may be time structured, for example, every week or biweekly, or the contract may be written that the consultant be on call to the group.

Regularly scheduled sessions will often deal with cases that staff will present in which the behavior of a patient is proving stressful to staff, and they need further understanding of the patient. The more the dynamics of the patient's behavior are discussed, the better position the staff will be in to determine appropriate nursing or medical intervention. An example of a situation in which a group of nurses in a general hospital setting will request consultation involves the problem of evaluating family behavior. In one situation, a patient was diagnosed as having terminal cancer. The wife of the patient did not want him to know his diagnosis, although the nurses were sure that subconsciously he did. There was conflict over how to deal with the patient and how to help the wife. The consultant, in this case, helped staff to deal with their own feelings and then helped them devise a nursing plan of intervention for both patient and family.

Planned Change

Consultants are frequently contracted to aid in a planned change. For example, a general hospital plans an inpatient psychiatric service and engages a psychiatric consultant to help in the design, planning, and implemention of the program. Or change is planned for an existing program, for example, moving a psychiatric unit from a traditional medical model of care to an eclectic or human service focus. The consultant who contracts work for these situations should have a firm knowledge of the following:

How people are affected by change.

Factors that influence an individual's attitudes toward change.

How people react to change.

Predicting the extent of resistance.

Minimizing resistance to change.

A systematic approach to making change.

Planned change consultation also operates on the crisis principle—that is, disruption creates stress, and people are significantly affected by change.

Interdisciplinary Issues

A consultant may be contracted through an agency or hospital administration to consult in team meetings involving various disciplines. Consultants add their own insights and views to the issues being discussed. They also diagnose specific communication problems and may talk with staff separately about strategy in working with other disciplines. Most often issues discussed have crisis dimensions. For example, in one situation nurses were having difficulty communicating effectively with one physician who had patients who needed referral to other services such as social service. The referral was often not made because the nurse could not communicate with the physician (and he had to make the referral), or the physician did not agree with the need for referral. Another example is a case in which a patient had expressed a specific need to talk to the nurse about his condition and his feelings about dying, but the patient's physician forbade the nurses to meet the need and allow the patient to talk about his concerns. He wrote on the patient's chart, "Do not discuss patient's condition with him."

Staff Development

Very often the consultant will be contracted to aid in staff development by teaching specific concepts and interventions. This kind of consultation is noncrisis in focus and increases the consultee's knowledge about a case or specific problem. In such situations, the consultant functions as a specialist and his intention is to increase the consultees' knowledge.[2] Examples of such topics may be assessment, diagnosis, intervention of unresolved grief; management of the suicidal, alcoholic, or drug abuse patient; and other mental health issues.

The consultation in which didactic material is presented is usually structured. Teaching conferences may also be utilized. In the following case, the consultant responded to the staff's request for aid in making a decision about a patients' disposition by

[2] Ibid, pp. 149–154.

interviewing the patient before the group. Then the staff determined the plan of action with the nursing consultant.

> The staff at a Halfway House were discussing a series of crises that had occurred over a period of days. Over the weekend several friends of one of the patients were visiting the House. After the visitors left, several patients were missing money and their medications. One of the patients was suspected. Monday night after repeatedly being told not to be in the male dorm, the same female patient was found in the dorm. Since she had broken the rules of the House, it was recommended that she leave the House. She was told that her behavior was too disruptive for the rest of the patients to deal with and that she was unable to control her behavior. On Tuesday night this patient tried to jump out of the second-floor window. Another patient was able to hold her back. The staff requested consultation to determine the seriousness of the suicidal gesture and the method of dealing with this person in relation to House rules and regulations.

The consultant interviewed the patient with the staff present for two reasons: to teach interviewing techniques in this particular situation and to include the patient's request in the decision that the staff was to make about her staying or leaving the Halfway House.

Community Development

The preceding situations have applied to a mental health professional who contracts for a specific consultation situation. In a community mental health center, consultation may be part of the job description for staff. We now discuss consultation from that perspective.

Single request. A member from a community group may request consultation from the community mental health center about a particular situation. In one case, a town aide who worked with a religious group that provided mental health services to its congregation presented the following problem to the consultant:

> . . . What am I going to do? I have a woman who just came to me and she doesn't know what to do. Her husband is 80 years old, and he is beating her with his cane. He will not take his medications, and his wife wants to commit him to the state hospital.

In this situation the consultant suggested that the aide check the husband's record from the mental health center for any clues and also to find out what may have precipitated this new behavior in the home environment; that is, why the man was not taking his medications and what the wife really wanted. The aide found out that 3 years previously the husband was diagnosed with "early senility" and that the wife did not want him out of the home. The consultant suggested to the aide that the wife tell the husband that his behavior was upsetting, that she could not tolerate it, and that he had to take his medicine or else the police would have to come as they did 3 years before. The aide followed through with the recommendation. The result was positive. Once the wife was able to set the limit with the husband, he began taking his medicines again and the wife was able to manage him in the home. This prevented a psychiatric hospitalization. The consultation aided the community worker in providing direct services while the nursing consultant provided the indirect services of supervising the mental health worker.

Developing resources. A second kind of community consultation helps people develop and strengthen the mental health resources within their own community. One example would be helping a community organize an education program on sex education for the school system. In one situation the community mental health consultant held a workshop designed to teach leadership development to give the women in the community self-confidence in developing their own programs. The women met with the consultant as leader and talked of the changing role of women in society. These discussions led to the development of a women's center, which in turn led to the development of day care programs. As the women became more organized, the consultant decreased her input to the group, but she kept the interest alive and remained the catylist in bringing the women together. The consultant knew the community and knew what agencies to work with, for example, Community Action Group, Committee for Human Services, and other such groups. Knowing the community helps the consultant determine which services need to be provided.

Outreach workers. Outreach workers in community groups often consult with mental health professionals. Here, the consultant listens to the workers talk about their concerns with multiple problem families. The consultant primarily asks such questions as,

"Where do you see any possibilities with this family?" and helps the workers sort out the strengths of a family and helps them to be more objective in their work. This consultation is an indirect service to help redefine the client situation and to provide additional support to outreach workers.

THE CONSULTATION PROCESS

Contract

The first step in the consultation process is to establish the contract between the consultant and the consultee. Caplan emphasizes that in planning a consultation service, there must be an organization structure to provide a channel of communication between the potential consultees and their institution on the one hand, and the consultant on the other.[3]

Usually there is a request for services from the consultee. There may or may not be issues for negotiation. After the request is made, the consultant identifies what can be provided in terms of direct and indirect services. When this is agreed upon, the contract is signed. The contract should always be in writing if there is a fee or payment for services. In the case of the community mental health centers, consultation could be part of the regular job description, and thus there would be no fee.

The consultant should identify areas of responsibility. These usually include services to be provided, periodic reports evaluating the consultation, and the time allocation. It is essential that consultants know to whom they are accountable. If consultants intend to use their work with consultees for publication or for research purposes, this point must be clearly specified in the contract, and written permission must be given by the consultees.

Model for Consultation

In contracts between the consultant and consultee, the model used most commonly is face-to-face meetings. The request may change each meeting, or the consultant and consultee may work together on a problem over an extended period of time.

Media. Media are playing increasing roles in consultation in locations that are inaccessible to direct services. For example, there

---

[3] Ibid, p. 120.

is a television communication system between Massachusetts General Hospital and the health service at Boston's Logan Airport. This system aids in diagnosis.

Consultation may be provided by written communication or by telephone. Professionals often use the telephone to ask colleagues their opinions. Because of the increasing use of telephone consultation, it is recommended that all conversations be verified in duplicate for the consultant's records. For example, if litigation develops and the consultee said that his consultation provided information on a certain kind of intervention, the consultant needs to verify this conversation in court.

Case conference. The case conference includes several people and is generally led by the consultant. There are many advantages to group consultation. They have been outlined as follows by Gerald Caplan:[4]

1. Consultant's communications are received not only by the stable group members but by transients as well.
2. Peer group support strengthens the staff vis-à-vis the consultant and facilitates a nonhierarchical relationship.
3. Staff can benefit from the cognitive and emotional contributions of each other.
4. The more experienced staff can contribute information about the realities and possibilities of the specific disciplines' role than the consultant may be familiar with.
5. Less experienced staff can direct attention to the problems that may be obscured among the senior staff caused by stereotypes, defenses, blind spots, prejudices, frustrations. The issues can then be freed-up for group discussion.
6. Common theme distortions can be dealt with as group issues.

Case Insight

The consultee needs assistance in understanding the nature and implications of the client's difficulties and the factors in his environment initiating or perpetuating the difficulty. Understanding the client's situation will enable consultees to use their usual professional skills and resources. For example, in the cases of sexual child abuse, the offender may be a neighbor, and his presence is perpetuating the crisis. The consultant may suggest a family treatment situation to provide additional data on how to proceed in helping the child.

[4] Gerald Caplan, *Principles of Preventive Psychiatry* (New York: Basic Books, Inc. 1963), p. 212–31.

Action

The consultee needs to develop additional skills or develop appropriate facilities within the institution. Caplan states that one type of skill which consultants will be called upon to help consultees develop is a better use of self in the clinical setting.[5] The technique utilized by the consultant is to help the consultee work out a specific plan of action, such as developing new skills or communicating with other agencies or setting up a referral system. For example, consultation with police officers may focus on helping them strengthen their interviewing skills.

Identify the Consultee Crisis

The client's problem may have triggered an emotional reaction in the consultee, which will prevent the professional from being therapeutic. The consultee's perception of the client may be biased. For example, working with young dying patients may trigger feelings of identification in the nursing staff.

Social System Issues

Problems that are identified as being produced in the social system of the consultee will usually require consultation on organization, policy, and program planning. One example would be initiating new programs such as victim counseling within an emergency room of a general hospital.

The consultant must study the system involved and its characteristics. Dr. Charles Ferguson[6] speaks of the nature of human systems, their subsystems, their relationships, and what is required for effective functioning. He describes the system as always attempting to stabilize through "mutually effective interdependence of its parts." Examples of subsystems within a hospital are medicine, nursing, psychology, and social service. Consultants need to understand the nature and function of these subsystems. Ferguson[7] defines one function of a consultant as listening to "identify strain, misunderstandings, disrespect; in short, trouble between people who need a high degree of collaboration in their relationship." In addition, the consultant must always analyze what the attachment of a new person to an existing system means to that

[5] Gerald Caplan, *Concepts of Mental Health and Consultation,* p. 207.

[6] Charles K. Ferguson, "Concerning the Nature of Human Systems and the Consultant's Role," *J. of Applied Behav. Sciences* 4, No. 2 (1968), pp. 179–194.

[7] Ibid.

system. Does the consultant threaten the total system? How much risk is involved if the consultant is to be only a temporary member of the subsystem, leaving the ongoing change process to the subsystem?

In one situation the consultant heard that the director of an adjunct service had reacted negatively to the former consultant. While the new consultant was working within the system, she quickly picked up the director's negative feelings. The consultant was advised by the director of nurses who had contracted for her services to proceed without worrying about this director, for what the consultant would be doing was within the realm of nursing. Problems and conflicts continued, but this was the strategy that the consultee requested.

Style of Consultation

Consultants, depending on their personality style as well as their model of consultation, will use a variety of techniques in the process. Examples of such techniques are teaching and presenting didactic content, providing support to decision-making issues, acting as role model, clarifying issues and concerns, clarifying misunderstandings, intervening in group conflict, facilitating communication between community groups and services, and increasing the objectivity of a situation. The consultant may use one particular technique such as facilitating group problem-solving or increasing objectivity by theme interference, a technique described by Caplan.[8] Consultants are responsible for deciding which technique or combination of techniques is useful to the individual situation and for performing that technique not only as they see the need but as they have the expertise to carry it out. For example, to perform theme interference, the consultant must have a good understanding of psychoanalytic theory—in order to diagnose the theme and to intervene effectively. Not all consultants have the necessary background. If the consultant does not have some understanding of group dynamics, it would be risky to attempt to intervene in group conflict, even though the conflict may clearly be the barrier for effective functioning. The consultant functions in a variety of roles and must excel at choosing the appropriate role or combination of roles. In summary, the consultant may be teacher, coordinator, mediator, supervisor, clinician, facilitator, and role model.

[8] Gerald Caplan, *Principles of Preventive Psychiatry*, p. 247.

Entry

A prime responsibility of the consultant is to build an emotional bond with the consultee and to constantly be aware of its state. Caplan advises that the continuing link between consultee and consultant is provided by the strength of the relationship that develops between them.[9]

A major step in consultation is the entry of the consultant into the system. Much of the transition has to do with how the consultant has been presented to the consultees and how the consultees react to this. It is important to remember that anxiety holds the consultee in contact with the consultant and that it is the binding force. Thus, anxiety should not necessarily be reduced. Rather than reassuring the consultee that things will work out, Caplan suggests statements such as: "This is something I think we really should be anxious about. I should like to help you with the problem."[10]

Introductions are extremely important. For example, in one situation, a consultant was introduced as Miss X who was taking over the functions of Miss Y who had consulted to the service for the previous year. This introduction automatically set up barriers for the entry process. At the time, the new consultant was not aware of the former consultant's method of consulting. It soon became apparent that each consultant used different techniques. This difference in style had to be fully explored before the consultant could begin to build a relationship with the service. For example, the consultant soon learned that the nurses had utilized the former consultant as a clinician who would become involved with the "difficult" patients. They valued this function greatly. Furthermore, it became immediately apparent that the nurses had not adequately terminated their relationship with the consultant. They spoke of her in glowing terms and with a great deal of sadness. One nurse even said after the new consultant had finished explaining her function, "I'm so glad you're back."

Clarification of Role

In the early entry phase much time must be spent in clarifying one's role. It must be emphasized that consultation is a process that helps staff with specific problems of management and plan-

---

[9] Gerald Caplan, *Concepts of Mental Health and Consultation,* p. 122.
[10] Ibid, p. 123.

ning for patients, as well as increasing the knowledge and skills of the staff. The consultant must clarify role, model, and style of consultation, as well as be certain that the consultees are requesting these services.

Role model. The mental health consultant serves as a role model in (1) assessment, that is, looking at behavior rather than the medical diagnosis to assess a patient's emotional needs; (2) making use of all knowledge available from all sources to be sure that all data have been collected; (3) communicating with others so that all knowledge is known; (4) demonstrating an empathetic attitude toward patients; and (5) acknowledging one's own limitations when necessary.

As role model in the area of assessment, the consultant constantly asks for information to "fill the gaps," especially if she believes that the information is available. The consultant clarifies statements that are crucial to the problem being studied and makes linkages between facts that would most readily lead to the solution of the problem. To counteract dependency, the consultant encourages each one to offer his or her thoughts and solutions and specifically utilizes the data provided by the staff rather than introducing *psychiatric formulations* to blur the issue further. When staff indirectly offers insights or solutions, the consultant picks them up and says, "You seem to be suggesting . . ." or "I hear you saying . . . ." The consultant then can add in nonjargon terms a more direct interpretation, which the staff member can agree to and still call his own.

The role of resource person, interpreter of behavior, and demonstrator of techniques is important in consultation. The consultant demonstrates suggestions to deal with behavior by saying, "A nurse might say," or "You can say something like this in your own words . . . ."

SPECIFIC TECHNIQUES

Assessment

A major task is to assess the meaning of the client's problem in terms of emotional life of the consultee and of the institution. Such information and data comes from observing behavior of the consultee, looking for interpersonal clues, environmental pressures, and one's own reaction in listening to content.

Maintenance of the Relationship

The manner in which a positive relationship is built between consultant and consultee is dependent on the consultant's expressed attitude to the consultee. It is very important to show respect as one professional to another. Building relationships means accepting to some extent the role assigned to you whether or not you like it. For example, if you are called to consult to a group of school teachers, you may be expected to lecture to the teachers. Caplan states the importance of entering the system in the role assigned.[11]

Ego-Supportive Techniques

This technique is similar to the supportive aspect of any therapeutic relationship. As the consultee becomes less anxious and more confident in his abilities and skills to handle the problem, you will see him cope more effectively with the problem.

Softening the Superego

Caplan refers to this technique as "relaxation of superego pressure."[12] It is important to encourage the consultee to express all the feelings and thoughts that have developed regarding the situation without the fear of judgment by the consultant. For example, in working with alcohol counselors, they need to express their thoughts and feelings about the drinking history that an alcoholic person may give and to which they may have a negative reaction. Unless this happens the counselor will not be effective in working with this person.

The technique is to talk about the problem in terms of the client (or alcoholic person, as in the previous example) *not* the problem of the consultee. The consultee is freer to talk in terms of the client's value system as opposed to his own. The consultant is then in a position to demonstrate a relaxed, humanistic approach. Thus, the consultee can identify with the consultant.

It is also useful for consultees to express and explore their feelings toward other professionals when these feelings interfere with performing necessary care. It also helps staff to separate out what is unique in their own specialty area. For example, nurses may talk about feelings of helplessness in being assertive when

---

[11] Ibid, pp. 123–124.
[12] Ibid, p. 137.

they deal with physicians over treatment regimens. In one case a 65-year-old man was in a terminal stage of care. He was with-drawn and angry whenever staff approached him. One nurse was able to talk with him and listen to his anger about dying and "losing control" of his life. The nurse believed that the man should be allowed more control in planning his care. The physician, with-out consulting the nurse or patient, made plans for him to be transferred to a nursing home. The patient was not told until the morning he was to leave. There was no time for him to express his feelings. The nurse felt helpless in approaching the physician after the orders and referral had already been made. Nursing staff said that the "floor was too busy to take time to go over the problem." It was important for the nurse to present her thoughts and feelings about the management of this case at a weekly meet-ing with the consultant.

Humanizing the Client

Caplan describes this technique as the crux of the whole con-sultation process and labels the technique as "dissipating the stereotype."[13] He further emphasizes that this technical maneuver is possible only after the consultation relationship has been prop-erly developed, and the consultant is established as a role model. The timing of this technique is very important.

At the right time, the consultant helps the consultee see the client as a human being with thoughts and feelings and a reason for behaving as he does in the difficult situation under discussion. Ideally, the client can now be viewed in a new perspective as a human being who is capable of interaction and negotiation. This new view exposes the consultee to different and more productive ways in which he can deal with the client.

Termination

The model of consultation continues more or less according to the consultant's stated objectives, model, and style. However, the issue of termination of services should always be explicit. The prescribed time limit must be stated at the entry point, and the issue of termination should be brought up for discussion several sessions prior to the last one. Generally, consultation is termina-ted when the problems associated with the individual crisis have been resolved. Caplan suggests that the termination need not be final; rather, it should be regarded as an interruption in a chain.

[13] Ibid, p. 138.

He states, "The channel of communication should be left open, so that when further trouble arises, as it is likely to do, the contact can be renewed."[14]

The consultation period must be reviewed in terms of progress made as well as in terms of problems encountered. This is the cognitive evaluation. Feelings of the consultee about the process are also an essential part of termination, and evaluation and discussion of this completes the total experience for the consultee.

DIFFICULTIES IN THE
CONSULTATION PROCESS

Consultation is a human process and as such is subject to as many problem situations as any other therapeutic encounter. Consultants entering a system will anticipate many varied reactions. Sometimes consultants will reenter a system in which they have previously worked. If the consultant is in the same profession as the consultees, judgmental feelings may arise within the consultant, especially if there is resistance. The consultant must constantly work at making objective observations and at exploring the reasons for the feelings of anger and frustration in order to remedy the difficulty.

Fantasies

A potential difficulty involves the consultees' fantasies about the consultant. The consultant must recognize this human factor and constantly deal with it. Usually, these fears and fantasies are expressed implicitly. For example, in one situation, one very articulate and spontaneous nurse made the comment to a consultant that the consultent seemed "too normal to be in the psychiatric business." Further exploration of this statement revealed that the nurse thought that all mental health staff were a "little crazy."

Other fears and fantasies involve thoughts that the consultant may be evaluating the competence of the staff. Often this potential stall is corrected by the consultant's clearly identifying the objectives of the consultation and discussing the issue of confidentiality. Staff must know how much and to whom the content of the sessions will be made available.

Systems Problems

Problems may often occur because of the system and its operation rather than because of the consultees' problems. For example, communication and respect between subsystems may be

[14] Ibid, p. 127.

lacking. Mechanisms may be needed to correct communication problems. If the problem involves status issues between subsystems, for example, how medicine views nursing or how nursing views social work, we suggest that consultation be provided to the total system rather than to the one subsystem that feels that it is of lower status.

The issue of change within a subsystem may create a problem. How much change can take place within one subsystem if the change is going to be a threat to the status of the other subsystem may be a serious problem. For example, if the nursing subsystem were to become more independent of the total hospital system, an and especially from the medical subsystem, would conflicts be intensified to an intolerable degree?

More and more issues will concern the consultants the longer they remain consultants to the system. They often become the outlets for many of the staff's feelings of frustration. This outpouring of emotion may be a burden to the consultant if there is inadequate opportunity for resolution. Consultants are constantly making diagnoses of the staff's complaints and feelings. They must identify the complaints that are part of the role process and the complaints that are part of the system process.

SUMMARY

This chapter presents a brief introduction to the process of mental health consultation. Mental health professionals are called upon to provide consultation as work in the community expands. Clinicians are called upon to consult within subsystems of the health care delivery system. This chapter identifies some basic issues in consultation: how requests for consultation are made, the consultation process itself; and problems in the consultation process.

II

target populations

The second part of the book deals with target population groups that frequently come to the attention of the mental health professional and are in the community, but that should be more carefully identified. Two groups of people who may easily be neglected by clinicians are the bereaved who are suffering from unresolved grief and the infertile couple. Three population groups who are always in the clinician's awareness, but for whom treatment models are difficult to implement include the alcoholic, the drug abuser, and the suicidal patient. Patient populations that have neither been treated properly nor adequately acknowledged as deserving treatment are victims and families of major crimes of homicide, rape, and attempted kidnapping; the aggressive sexual offender; and the prostitute.

6
the bereaved

Virtually everyone must deal with grief some time in his or her lifetime. These grief reactions may follow the death of grandparents, parents, siblings, children, friends, national leaders, or celebrities. Some people also appear to experience the process of grief following events in which a person has not died. These include knowledge of one's own impending death, abortions, separations, divorce, aging in loved ones, loss of children's dependence, alterations of body image (through aging, surgery, wearing dental braces or glasses, growing bald, losing teeth), leaving a familiar neighborhood, giving up a life's dream, "giving up" neurotic behavior, and even finishing a good book.

Most people are able to normally experience the grief process, and no information exists as to the percentage of people who experience pathological grief. From a clinical perspective, however, it has been our experience that in 10 to 15 percent of patients that request outpatient treatment, pathological grief plays a central role in their psychopathology.

The most common reaction to pathological grief is a mild, chronic depression. In most instances this reaction is hardly noticeable. The person may withdraw from friends, stop going to church, feel guilty in various situations, and suffer various aches and pains. More severe reactions to failure to grieve include severe depression, schizophrenic reactions, psychosomatic disorders, or acting out behavior. Under the stress of unresolved grief, the person will regress according to his vulnerability.

THE PROCESS OF NORMAL GRIEF

In order to understand pathological grief and its impact on people in the community, it is important to describe the process of normal grief.

Grief is a psychological process following a loss, which allows one to cope in a gradual manner with an overwhelming loss so that it can be accepted as a reality. If the full impact of the loss were suddenly experienced, the person might be psychologically overwhelmed. In grief the existence of the one who is lost is prolonged so that the person gradually may come to terms with what has happened.

The initial reactions to learning of the loss are shock and disbelief. "It just could not have happened. I don't believe it." The denial of the event is illustrated by the expectation on the part of the bereaved that the lost person will appear or that the voice of the dead person will be heard in the next room.

The bereaved experiences painful feelings of sadness and emptiness as he recalls the lost person. The psychological discomfort is often accompanied by waves of weeping, experiencing a feeling of tightness in the throat, or a choking accompanied by a shortness of breath and sighing. Feelings of exhaustion are common. These waves or pangs of grief occur less frequently as time goes on but may be readily reawakened when memories of the lost person are recalled.

The bereaved is preoccupied with the image of the deceased, and he reviews and relives many of the memories involving the lost person as if to put the memories and the dead person to rest once and for all.

In the early phases of grief the bereaved often feels guilty. "Maybe there was something I could or should have done." There may be guilt for being the survivor, for not doing enough, or for never making peace with the dead.

The bereaved tends to be irritable and angry. Sometimes the anger is directed toward the dead person for not remaining alive, for leaving work unfinished, and for causing all the grief.

In normal grief the bereaved eventually frees himself from certain ties to the deceased by acknowledging and bearing the pain of the loss, by experiencing the feeling of sadness, and by recalling memories involving the deceased. When these tasks are successfully handled, the acute phase of normal grief lasts from 2 weeks to 2 months. Signs and symptoms of grief, however, may last for as long as one year. Establishing new relationships and interests, the ability to function as before the loss, and renewed capacity for pleasure are signs of the resolution of the grief.

Parkes,[1] in his excellent book on bereavement, summarizes major aspects of grieving according to the following seven features:

1. A process of realization, i.e. the way in which the bereaved person moves from denial or avoidance of recognition of the loss towards acceptance.
2. An alarm reaction—anxiety, restlessness, and the physiological accompaniments of fear.
3. An urge to search for and to find the lost person in some form.
4. Anger and guilt, including outbursts directed against those who press the bereaved person towards premature acceptance of his loss.
5. Feelings of internal loss of self or mutilation.
6. Internalization phenomena—the adaption of traits, mannerisms, or symptoms of the lost person, with or without a sense of his presence within the self.
7. Pathological variants of grief, i.e., the reaction may be excessive and prolonged or inhibited and inclined to emerge in distorted form.

Grief as a Social Process

Grief is a social process because it can best be handled when it is shared and assisted by others. Few people seem to be able to grieve entirely alone.

Various cultures and religions recognize grief as a social process and provide religious and social rules of conduct that assist the bereaved. These rules state who shall be with the bereaved before the burial, who shall say what during the burial, and the duration and kind of social interaction after the burial. The rules of conduct further describe on what anniversaries or religious holidays the bereaved will again meet with others to remember his loss.

[1] Colin Murray Parkes, *Bereavement: Studies of Grief in Adult Life* New York: (International Universities Press, Inc., 1972)

For example, in Orthodox Judaism, after the initial period of grief, families go to the temple twice a day for eleven months to pray. Then four times a year they attend memorial services.

In the Irish culture the wake prior to the funeral is a time for the sharing of grief through the viewing of the body, lamenting, and paying tribute through eulogies. The wake is frequently portrayed in song and story.

It becomes even more evident that grief is a social process when we view the rapid changes developing in contemporary society that are making it even more difficult for people to grieve.

1. As a result of technology, we are a mobile people without roots. 30 percent of our population moves each year. Consequently, people who suffer a loss are likely to be far from the relatives and old friends who would be in the best position to help with the process of grieving. We have observed that people who are isolated from friends and relatives will seek out professionals (nurses, family physicians, psychiatrists) for assistance with their normal grief.

2. The "religious" rules of conduct used traditionally for handling the process of grief are losing their importance because of the diminishing impact of religion in our culture. This is unfortunate as (religion aside) these rules comprise a wealth of psychological wisdom that our society can ill afford to lose.

3. The process of grief may also be obstructed because of hospitalization and medical technology. With people dying in hospital rooms and intensive care units rather than in the home, family are excluded or frightened away so that the process of dying is made into something unnatural and unreal. This inevitably hinders the normal grief process.

4. The growth of cities and the scarcity of space have resulted in overcrowded cemeteries that are, of necessity, difficult to reach and unappealing to visit. Some cemeteries have even been moved to make room for highways. In vanishing rural America the cemetery often occupies a scenic hill where children and adults may easily visit. Under these conditions, death is more likely to be seen as a natural part of the life cycle.

5. Because of the increased liberality of the abortion laws, with a total increase in abortions, there is an increased need to grieve. For many women the abortion represents a loss that must be dealt with psychologically. If the demand for abortions leads to impersonal procedures that ignore psychological needs, we may see pathological reactions arising from the failure to grieve.

Society will continue to change at an ever-increasing rate, and change will lead to psycho-social problems. Society may find new solutions to the problems created by change—but until it does, there will be psychological "casualties." We believe that the normal grieving process is one of the casualties of change. By understanding the social and psychological process of grief, one can have an important impact on large numbers of patients.

The ultimate impact on a person as a result of a loss of a loved one must also be viewed in social terms. For many, there is a deprivation of status, role, income, companionship, and sexual activity that may be irreplaceable. A 65-year-old childless widow recently told of her missing the pleasure in having nightly sexual intercourse with her husband for the entire 40 years of their marriage. She knew that in spite of her "successful grieving" it was highly unlikely that she would ever recapture this pleasure.

Many widows and widowers lack the ability to replace for themselves that which has been deprived. At the same time, they are discriminated against by society from achieving for themselves what they need and want. Parkes applies the term *stigma*, or change in attitude towards the widow, as the reason leading to her social isolation.

WHY PEOPLE FAIL TO GRIEVE

We find it useful for the purpose of therapy to classify the causes of failure to grieve (or pathological grief) into social and psychological factors.

Social Factors: The Absence of a Supportive Social System

Social negation of a loss. Pathological grief may result from situations in which the loss is not socially defined as such. This may occur following an abortion where the expectation is either that the person will keep the event a secret or that the woman should be grateful that the procedure is completed. The situation may be further complicated by the anger directed towards the woman for being "careless," and for inconveniencing others. Similar dynamics occur when a woman gives up an infant for adoption. With both adoption and abortion, there is the task of grieving to be done, but the social support necessary for the process is often inadequate.

Because of the number of patients who present for help following abortion or giving up a child, we routinely inquire about these possibilities in all women of child-bearing age. The diagnosis is more certain when the presentation for help occurs, as it often does, on the anniversary of the loss.

A socially unspeakable loss. Pathological grief may result when the loss is so "unspeakable" that those members in the social system of the bereaved cannot be of any help. As an example, a 24-year-old, bright, attractive young woman was found dead from an overdose of morphine. There was no prior history of drug abuse. It was never determined whether the death resulted from foul play, accident, or suicide. Because of the uncertainty, no one would ask the bereaved mother the usual questions that facilitate the grieving process such as, "When did it happen? " "Where did it happen?" "How did it happen?" The mother failed to grieve and made a suicide attempt one month after the funeral in an attempt to "join my daughter." Following the suicide attempt, the patient was referred to a psychiatrist with whom the loss could be discussed. The patient was able to grieve successfully in ten weekly visits.

Geographic distance from social support. Pathological grief may occur if the person is away from his social supports at the time of mourning. In one situation, a mother decided not to tell her 20-year-old daughter of the father's death until college examinations were completed. By the time the daughter returned home, the family had completed their grieving. They were perplexed over the daughter's tears and provided little in the way of support for her grief. She sought psychiatric help the following year.

In other situations where the person is informed of the death, there may be social isolation from family as a result of geographic distance or psychological alienation. Some people have neither family nor close friends. It is hoped that they will seek help from clinics or mental health personnel.

Assuming the social role of the "strong one." Some people are designated the role of the "strong one" by those around them. In family situations, they are expected to make the arrangements for the funeral and be supportive to everyone else. Needless to say, these people miss the opportunity to deal with their own grief.

The "strong one" impasse also occurs outside of the family setting. In one situation, an operating room nurse was noted to be crying by her physician and nurse colleagues. They insisted that she go to the psychiatric clinic for "therapy" even though they knew that her best friend had been killed in an auto accident just two days before. Her social support system believed that operating room nurses—like Marines—are not supposed to cry.

Undertainty over the loss. In situations where the loss is uncertain, for example, the case in which the information is that "your husband is missing in action," both the wife as well as the social support system are unable to deal with the possible loss.

Psychological Factors

Where psychological factors predominate, a supportive social system alone will not resolve the grief.

Ambivalence towards the lost person. Pathological grief may occur when the person has profoundly ambivalent feelings—intense love and intense hate—towards the dead person. The person is frightened to grieve for fear of discovering the intensely negative and unacceptable feelings. Obsessional people with strict and rigid superego structures are apt to suffer from the above psychological dilemmas.

Overcathexis of the lost person. A person may be so dependent on or place such a high value on the dead person that he will not grieve so as to avoid the reality of the loss. One patient said: "Mother was half of my ego. I would not be complete without her. She cannot be dead."

Overwhelmed by multiple loss. Some people who experience multiple losses such as the death of an entire family have difficulty grieving on two counts. First, the loss is too overwhelming to contemplate. Second, the family who supports the grief is no longer available. A patient of the author (A.L.) experienced a multiple loss as a result of five miscarriages due to a uterine defect. In therapy, the patient grieved the loss of each fetus one at a time. The patient had a name and a set of hopes and dreams for each.

The need to be strong and in control. Some people do not permit themselves to grieve for fear of losing control or appearing weak, to themselves and to others. One patient said that if she began to cry, she feared the tears would never stop.

Reawakening an old loss. Some people are reluctant to grieve because the current loss reawakens a more painful loss that had not yet been dealt with. The death of a distant aunt, for instance, may reawaken the death of a mother which may have occurred years before.

THE DIAGNOSIS AND TREATMENT OF PATHOLOGICAL GRIEF

Diagnosis

The diagnosis of pathological grief may be inferred from the following historical data and interview observations:

1. If a patient fails to grieve following the death of a loved one, a diagnosis of pathological grief should be considered. The patient may not have cried, may have absented himself from the funeral, and may have put thoughts of the deceased out of his mind.
2. Pathological grief should be considered when the patient becomes symptomatic on the anniversary of a loss, when the symptoms recur the same time each year, or when symptoms occur during the holidays (especially Thanksgiving and Christmas).
3. Pathological grief should be considered when the patient avoids visiting the grave and refuses to participate in religious memorial services of loved ones when these practices are a part of the patient's culture.
4. Pathological grief should be considered when the patient develops a chronicity of normal grief symptoms, especially persistant guilt and lowered self-esteem.
5. Pathological grief should be considered when the patient continues to search for the lost person after a prolonged period of time. Some patients make the search while in fugue states. Others may wander from town to town and/or act as if they are expecting the dead one to return. They may even consider suicide to effect the reunion.
6. Pathological grief should be considered when a relatively minor event triggers off symptoms of grief. This event is psychodynamically connected to the original loss.
7. Pathological grief should be considered whenever a patient is unable to discuss someone who has died with relative equanimity. When the voice cracks and quivers and the eyes become moist, unresolved grief over the person in question is quite likely.
8. Pathological grief should be considered when an interview is characterized by themes of loss.
9. Pathological grief should be considered when the patient experiences bodily symptoms similar to those of the dead person after the normal period of grief.

10. Pathological grief should be considered when the patient's relationships to friends and relatives shifts for the worse following the death. This may represent a displacement of feelings from the dead person.

The Treatment of Unresolved Grief

In order for a delayed or incomplete grief reaction to be successfully treated, the person has to experience the feelings and thoughts that were initially avoided. He is likely to cry, to have detailed recollections of the dead person, to dream more actively of the dead person, and to reminisce. This process is often completed in 6 to 10 weeks. With a successful outcome, we have seen patients no longer have bodily aches that plagued them from the time of the loss. They experience positive and warm feelings towards the deceased, remembering them not as they were during their dying days and in the coffin but as they were in happier times. They experience a "sweet sadness" over the deceased, not a bitterness. One patient described a feeling, after completing the delayed grief, that the axe was now out of her heart. There is sometimes a feeling that time had resumed after "standing still" for the years since the loss had occurred. Two patients which the author (A.L.) treated commented that the New Year's Eve following the regrief work was very special. "I said goodbye 1974 and goodbye 1964 (the year of the loss)." After successful regrief work, people feel increased self esteem, less guilt, and may resume church affiliation, if that was their pattern prior to the loss. They begin to visit the cemetery. Relationships that had been compromised because of a displacement of feelings from the dead person are channeled in a healthier direction. One patient who failed to grieve a miscarriage of an 8-month female fetus had an extraordinary amount of difficulty relating to her next born daughter. After successfully dealing with the grief, the patient commented on how appealing and responsive her daughter had become.

How can one assist with the regrief process? Who can provide this assistance?

For the large numbers of people who fail to grieve because of the absence of an available and supportive social matrix, help can be easily provided. The therapeutic person needs only to gently encourage the patient to discuss the loss and then to bear with the bereaved during the grief process. He or she will be carefully but subtly scrutinized by the grieving person to see whether there is strength, respect, and kindness. It may be helpful to educate and reassure the person as to what is expected, what is all right. We reassure the bereaved, if necessary, that they will not cry forever, permanently lose control, or go crazy if they grieve. We have never seen these untoward consequences. To the contrary, these things may occur from a failure to grieve. If the person laments that the past is the past and should remain buried, we reply that the past is very much in the present because it has not really been buried. Grieving is necessary to put the past in its proper perspective.

For those people who experience considerable difficulty in grieving, especially those for whom there are psychological causes for failure to grieve, more active measures may be necessary. Special therapeutic skills may here be necessary. The clinician may help the bereaved reconstruct memories to elicit the feelings. "What did she look like?" "What happened the last time you talked with her?" "Where were you standing when you visited the hospital?" "Who else was in the room?"

When failure to grieve results from strongly ambivalent feelings towards the deceased, it is useful and necessary for the person to express the negative feelings. This must be encouraged, however, not by confrontation but by a gentle and supportive approach. For instance, the bereaved may be reassured by the clinician of the strength of the positive feelings that he knows exist. Only then may the patient be willing to verbalize the negative feelings. Sometimes it is easier to assist the bereaved to discuss "disappointments with" rather than "anger toward" the dead person. In discussing negative feelings, it is often easier for the bereaved to use words such as "irritation," "annoyance," or "aggravation," rather than "anger."

The bereaved will need to deal with multiple losses one at a time.

When there is an overcathexis toward the dead person, a firm therapeutic relationship may need to be established before the bereaved dares "give up" the dead person.

The overall response to regrief work is hard to predict. We have seen no one get worse. We have seen most people improve to varying degrees. In the most dramatic cases, we have seen people improve to their level of functioning before the death occurred, even if the event occurred 25 years before. In other situations, improvement is limited by pathological personalities that are not clearly apparent until the grief work is done.

In general, helping a person with regrief work can be a most gratifying experience for a clinician.

Case Illustration

Case history. A 53-year-old married mother of one became depressed and was hospitalized one week after her only child, a 21-year-old female, moved one block away to her own apartment. In addition to the classical depressive symptomotology, the patient was expressing hostility towards her daughter in a thinly veiled manner: "When my daughter hears how sick I am, I fear it will be the death of her."

The patient was an only child who had been living alone with her widowed mother at the time of the latter's death. The patient, who had a hostile dependent relationship on her mother, failed to grieve following the death. Shortly thereafter, she had met a man, married 6 months later, immediately become pregnant, and had a daughter whom she named after her dead mother. At the patient's insistence, the infant had remained in the hospital for 3 months because the patient feared she would harm her. This infant, now 21 years old, was about to leave home.

Formulation and treatment. The patient, unable to deal with her own ambivalence toward her mother, fails to grieve following her mother's death. She deals with some of her dependency needs by marrying and by producing a child who is the recipient of her mother's name, as well as the patient's feelings toward her mother. The daughter's leaving reawakens the patient's original loss of her mother. This precipitates a depression.

Treatment consisted of helping the patient grieve the loss of her mother. The patient was then able to make a psychological distinction between her daughter and her mother. This treatment allowed the patient to experience healthy mothering feelings towards the daughter and positive memories towards the mother. Most important, the depressive symptoms subsided, and the daughter was able to leave home.

7

the infertile couple

by Barbara Eck Menning, R.N., M.S.

A second population group that has been neglected by clinicians, both clinically and in the professional literature, is that containing the infertile people. A diagnosis of infertility has the potential to trigger a crisis reaction in the adult female or male. One of the tasks in adulthood is parenting. When this task is biologically denied, as through the diagnosis of infertility, the person is crisis prone. All health workers must understand the physiological, psychological, and social components involved in this developmental crisis in order to exercise a therapeutic effect in the helping process.

CONCEPT OF INFERTILITY

Infertility represents a complex life crisis to those involved. Emotionally stressful, financially expensive, psychologically threatening, and often physically painful, it is all the more so because it is rarely *expected*.

Barbara Eck Menning, R.N., M.S., is a nurse-educator specializing in maternal–child health. She is founder and director of *Resolve*, a Boston-based organization, which counsels infertile people.

Physicians define *infertility* as *the inability to conceive a pregnancy after one year of sexual relations without contraception or the inability to carry pregnancy to a live birth.* A couple should not be bound by an imposed definition of infertility. They have the right to ask to be considered "infertile" whenever they begin to feel that they are, especially if they are over 30 years of age or if either has had a fertility related event or disease (such as endometriosis or pelvic inflammatory disease in women or orchitis or varicocele in men, or venereal disease in either). It is also possible that single people may want to have their fertility status evaluated. For those who care greatly about having biological children, this is a reasonable request.

Infertility is frequently subdivided into *primary infertility*, which occurs without history of previous conception, and *secondary infertility*, which may occur after one or more successful pregnancies. The reasons for secondary infertility are many of the same as those for primary infertility. Each pregnancy is unique and tells nothing about the potential for a future pregnancy. Both kinds of infertility will be dealt with in this chapter as one.

It is estimated that 15 percent of the population of childbearing age in America is infertile at any given time. The three basic causes of infertility break down almost equally: male factor 35 percent, female factor 35 percent, and combined factor 30 percent. The general public is greatly misinformed about infertility and generally considers it a *female* disorder. Statistics, however, show that this is far from true. This is why both the woman and the man must be studied in a work-up or else the results will not be complete. The following case example illustrates this situation:

> Don was a successful businessman of 28 when he married. He and his wife June used birth control for 2 years while they established a comfortable home. June conceived the month after birth control was stopped. Unexpectedly, at 11 weeks of gestation, June experienced bleeding and cramping. She was hospitalized and lost the pregnancy. Following this episode, pregnancy did not occur again. After 1½ years the couple sought medical advice. June was worked up thoroughly and found to be normal. The doctor suggested that she quit her teaching position and try to "relax." After another year, the couple decided to seek another medical opinion. This doctor insisted that Don be examined as well as his wife. A semen analysis revealed a normal sperm count but very low motility. Medical treatment did not improve the condition. At this point Don and June have sought counseling prior to considering artificial insemination.

Even though the infertility rate is high—involving over 8½ million people in this country—the successful "cure rate," referring to those who achieve a pregnancy and live birth, is increasing steadily. Research and technology developed within the last 5 years have dramatically improved the diagnostic tools and treatment available to a physician. This new technology has been made possible, in part, by pressure on the medical profession to come up with better results, for adoption, the once easy alternative to biological parenthood, is no longer readily available. A competent specialist in infertility now cures between 50 and 60 percent of his patients. This is an optimistic note and should encourage infertile couples to pursue diagnosis and treatment. However, the rigorous tests and treatments now available are not without their psychic cost. It is possible that when couples submit to this regimen and do *not* become pregnant, they may arrive at the end in a state of emotional, physical, and financial exhaustion.

Infertility appears to be increasing in the population. There are many speculations as to why this might be so. Certainly, some sociological trends, such as delaying marriage and childbearing into the years after 30 and the prolonged use of birth control (particularly the pill and interuterine devices), might be partially responsible. Veneral disease is reaching epidemic levels in some parts of the country. If allowed to go untreated, it is a major threat to both male and female fertility. Some doctors now believe that the new abortion legislation and the resultant high abortion rate are beginning to be reflected in the infertility rate. It is possible that abortions performed under less than ideal conditions may be a source of subsequent infection and may result in infertility. It is also true that more accurate reporting and recording of health conditions will reflect a higher infertility rate.

DIAGNOSING INFERTILITY

Procedure

Diagnostic procedures may vary, depending on the physician selected or the clinic chosen. It is advised that a couple seek out a professional group which specializes in infertility, if it is available, as well as a physician in whom they have trust and in whom they can confide. The sequence of diagnostic procedures will vary, but it will include some or all of the following:

1. General physical examination and history of both man and woman.
2. Pelvic examination for the woman.

3. Interpretation of the basal temperature charts of the woman's cycles.
4. Semen analysis and possible further diagnostic tests, such as testicular biopsy, X-ray study of testicles, and vas deferens.
5. Post-coital test.
6. Tubal insufflation for the woman. Further study may include uterotubogram.
7. Endometrial biopsy.
8. Blood and urine studies.
9. Culdoscope or laparoscopy.

The nonpregnant woman is advised to see her gynecologist once a year for a pelvic and breast examination and Pap test. The woman who has infertility problems will probably see her specialist once a month or more during her diagnostic phase and perhaps even more often in the treatment phase. The man generally has fewer infertility tests to be performed and the time involved in the process is considerably less. Treatments performed on the man may be classified as "noninvasive" as opposed to the "invasive" examinations required for the female. Because of the nature of the examinations and tests, the concept of privacy becomes most important as a component of the rights of the patient. For example, it is an unpleasant and embarassing experience for a woman to remove her clothes and lie on a table with her feet in stirrups and to be draped with a sheet (for her privacy?) so that she cannot see what is being done to her. The doctor will probably be a man, for 93 percent of gynecologists are men.

The nurse, acting as a patient advocate in this situation, has a major responsibility in collaborating with the physician to ensure that the patient's rights are respected. The following list has been documented through discussion groups involving infertile people:

Patient's Rights

Initial appointment

1. The patient has the right to be seen, fully clothed, in the physician's office to discuss the case and ask questions *before* being examined. If this is the patient's first visit, this may be *all* she wants. It is important for the woman to determine if she and the physician are of the same philosophy and if a good rapport is possible. If not, she should seek another physician.
2. The patient has the right to be seen on time or to be given an indication of the approximate time wait. The patient's time is valuable.

3. The patient has the right to be treated respectfully and called one's full name. Interviewing and record taking should be done in privacy.

Physical examination

1. On the examining table the patient has the right to be draped in such a manner that she may see what is being done. Some physicians have special lights and mirrors so that a patient may participate fully and understand each test or treatment.
2. The patient has the right to have everything explained *before* the doctor begins. The doctor should tell why he is doing the procedure, if it will hurt, if there may be any possible side effects, and when any results will be known. The patient should be advised of the cost of any procedure, and the doctor should know the limits of his patient's insurance coverage.

   In one case example a woman was scheduled to have a tubal insufflation. The patient had no idea what results the physician and nurse were looking for, but she was very much aware that she was supposed to have some physical reaction when she was assisted to a sitting position on the examining table. The next day she had to attend a conference and was extremely uncomfortable with shoulder pain. However, she had not been informed what this might mean. Inadequate patient teaching only served to make the woman feel more anxious and tense about her infertility studies.
3. The patient has the right to be talked to in language she can understand. Women seem to have more difficulty with this issue then men. Doctors and nurses may be guilty of "taking down" to a patient or they may hide behind polysyllabic terms or abbreviations. Perhaps the worst violator is the doctor or nurse who says nothing at all about what diagnostic or treatment procedures are in progress. The nurse is an important person in helping the patient to understand what the doctor has said or done by specifically asking the patient what she understands and what she has questions about.
4. The patient has the right to know the name and dosage of any medication or solution given to her. She also has the right to know the name, amount, and reason for any specimen taken from her.
5. The patient has the right to know her vital signs and blood pressure if they are taken and the complete results of any specimens which have been taken (blood, urine, tissue, etc.)

Decisions on treatment

1. The patient in a teaching hospital or clinic is sometimes asked to participate in research studies or to be seen by students of the health professions. She has the right to refuse either. If she accepts, she should have careful explanations of everything that is done and should sign a form for any research project.

2. Decisions which affect the patient's body and health must ultimately be made by the patient (and her family). The doctor can only make recommendations. The patient has the right to ask for a second opinion before making important decisions.
3. The patient should not be asked to sign any consent forms or documents which have not been fully explained. She should never have to sign under pressure or duress.
4. The patient has the right to change doctors as often as necessary to locate a practitioner who treats her with respect and competence. The patient should always be able to obtain a summary of her record from a previous doctor by writing and requesting that it be sent to her next doctor. It is a patient's responsibility to write to her previous physician and inform him of her reason for leaving his practice or for seeking another opinion.

The issue of patient's rights is very important in the treatment of the infertile person. In many cases, the physician or nurse unwittingly violates the patient's rights because they wish to spare the woman needless worry over the facts and realities of her body. Women have supported this attitude for generations, saying such things as, "You're the doctor, you do what you think is best," or "Don't tell me what you are doing. I'd rather not know." Some women have great difficulty in challenging any male in an authority position because they have been taught to be polite and nice to people. Some doctors do not tell a patient that something is going to hurt because they fear that she will tense up or overreact. They may not tell a patient that a drug or treatment will have side effects for fear of "suggesting" it. Some doctors believe that a woman is truly comforted by a paternalistic "father–child" relationship with her doctor. Some use familiarity and joking to set the patient "at ease." Nevertheless, now that women are becoming more knowledgeable in all areas, including their own bodies, patient's rights require that adult patients be treated as adults. The doctor–patient relationship should be the same as any other service–consumer relationship.

A word about communications. The patient, it seems, invariably blames herself for not understanding medical words, tests, parts of the anatomy, names of medications, and so on. Patients should be encouraged to become as familiar with their bodies and functions as possible. Beyond that, it is the responsibility of the doctor or nurse to explain and to interpret words at the level of the patient's understanding. Health professionals are taught communication skills, but all too often they are forgotten or discarded. The patient who is under high anxiety or emotional stress hears and perceives *selectively* and may even have partial or total memory lapse about the conversation. The doctor and nurse must repeat important points several times, and they should ask the patient to repeat what she has heard. Remember:. *What the doctor or nurse says is only half the communication. What the patient hears and understands is the more important half.*

PSYCHOLOGICAL COMPONENTS

Feelings about Infertility

The psychological components of infertility are many and very real. People confronting such a diagnosis find that they experience varying feeling states. Not all people feel emotional pain of equal intensity, but most can express feelings and emotions which are particularly difficult to bear.

Surprise. The first feeling, although temporary and superficial, is one of surprise. Most people generally assume that they are fertile. And one cannot, obviously, know if one is fertile until one attempts to become pregnant. Many infertile couples give histories of using birth control for many years. It is not until the couple try to conceive a child that the problem becomes conscious and reality based.

Isolation. As the awareness of infertility grows on a couple, a feeling of isolation and loneliness often occurs. This is a personal and inherently sexual problem. It is not easy to talk about. Family and friends usually keep an embarrassed distance from the subject or else they offer platitudes, misinformation, or gratuitous psychiatric advice. "Relax!" "Take a second honeymoon!" If the wife works, "Quit!" If she is staying at home, "Get a job!" Little wonder that a couple may keep their feelings very much to themselves. In the process, they may lean so heavily upon each other that marital stress results. The following is one such example:

Betty had a therapeutic abortion at age 20 for a premarital pregnancy. She married another man 2 years later and used birth control for a year while she finished a graduate course. When she failed to conceive after being off birth control for 6 months, Betty became very anxious and sought medical care. Her husband was found to be normal, but Betty had moderate adhesions of both Fallopian tubes. She underwent tuboplasty which appeared to improve her situation. Still no pregnancy resulted. Betty's anxiety over her infertility increased, and she found herself unable to work (which involved small children). Her relationship with her husband deteriorated into frequent fights and talk of divorce. Betty sought therapy as a last resort. She felt almost immediate improvement when she was helped to express unresolved feelings about her abortion. As she experienced and acknowledged feelings of guilt and grief, she found her present infertility more bearable. She and her husband have reconciled and Betty has resumed her work. They are seriously considering remaining childfree.

Anger. When a couple enter a diagnosis and attempted treatment of infertility, they surrender much control of their bodies and destinies to the care of the physician who treats them. Even in the best of medical relationships, the feelings of helplessness are extreme. At this point anger is often displayed. The anger is often very rational—focused at real and correctly perceived insults, such as pressure from familes to "produce" or the pain and stress of various tests or treatments. Some anger may be irrational—displaced onto targets such as the physician or the adoption agency, but it is really a result of the abject helplessness that the couple feel.

Grief. When it is diagnosed that pregnancy will be impossible for a couple, the necessary and unavoidable feeling which must be experienced is *grief*. To deny or repress this feeling will prolong the resolution process indefinitely. The grief usually runs the classic course of shock, suffering, and recovery. Each person goes through these stages in his own way and at his own speed. One very real barrier to the expression of this sense of grief is that family and friends of the infertile couple are not always aware of the situation, and even if they are, they may not understand that a loss has occurred. The loss in this case is of a *potential*, not actual, child, but the feelings are often as intense as if an actual death had occurred. The couple themselves may not realize that they have important grief work to do. In desperation, they may turn to immediate plans of adopting children or of heroically espousing the childfree life. The underlying feelings may linger indefinitely as feelings of depression, lassitude, and inability to direct thoughts persist. It is a complicating factor when a couple proceed to adopt a child or children before they have settled their grief over infertility. By ignoring or suppressing feelings, couples may inadvertently affect the quality of their relationships with their adopted children for years to come. This is one reason that adoption workers ask the couple personal and pointed questions when they are doing a home study. They attempt to assess to what degree the couple have resolved the issue of infertility.

Standing alone. The literature often talks of an "infertile couple," but when the final word is given, unless it is a combined biophysiological problem, one person stands alone for a time and realizes that he or she is the person with the infertility problem and that he or she is denying the marriage partner genetic children. The infertile partner may entertain fears or fantasies that the fertile partner will leave, or worse, stay and be secretly hostile and condemning. There may be a period of turmoil in which the infertile partner behaves erratically and attempts to prod the other partner into revealing the perceived negative feelings. This "begging the question" usually culminates in an admission by the fertile partner that they are *both* hurt and disappointed by the turn of events. This simple disclosure seems to lay the blame and guilt away and allows the couple to get on with the business of living.

There are few health conditions as threatening to one's sexuality as infertility. A man who is infertile seems to suffer keenly in his concept of masculinity or virility. This is especially true when the problem is a low or absent sperm count. The process of being "counted or scored" is intensely disturbing and threatening to many men. Men also react with similar feelings when the problem is related to inability in deposition of sperm because of anatomical abnormalities, impotence, or premature ejaculation. When the problem is one of low motility or blockage in the transport of sperm, the man may accept his problem with more equanimity. Such problems are usually acquired and have no congenital or psychogenic origins. More important, they leave the highly-charged issue of sperm production and ability to perform intercourse intact.

Women are also affected by infertility in their sense of sexuality. If the woman had a traditional upbringing, she may have defined her entire sexuality, or even her entire identity, around childbearing. When this is denied her, she must reexamine her concept of sexuality and attempt to redefine it around the fact that childbearing will not occur. It is important for her to see that she is neither defective nor impaired nor less than whole because she does not complete this one potential. Infertile women are often able to learn this important lesson when they talk with women who have no desire to bear children, women who choose to remain celibate, and women past the childbearing age who are self-actualizing. In RESOLVE, a Boston-based organization which counsels infertile people, men and women have the opportunity to come together with other infertile people and discover their feelings about sexuality and work toward resolution.

Women, more than men, seem to mourn the loss of the childbearing experience per se. Many women specifically grieve over the inability to see their bodies grow and change with pregnancy and to successfully master the labor and delivery of a child. These events are often highly idealized and may be the subject of dreams or fantasies. It is particularly true of women who have lost pregnancies through spontaneous or induced abortion that successful mastery of pregnancy and childbirth is important. Men, however, seem to mourn the loss of the child itself, and they often focus on aspects of the genetic heritage which is ended.

Surgical removal of any or all of the organs of reproduction may precipitate a double-edged grief process. The person needs to grieve the loss of her organs and regain an intact body image, as well as to grieve the loss of potential childbearing. The trade-off in these cases is usually that the surgery has been done to halt some life threatening or incapacitating condition and that the individual may usually find comfort in the reality of improved general health.

THE "NORMAL INFERTILE" COUPLE

In the words of one noted infertility specialist, "There is no such thing as a normal infertile couple. If they were normal, they wouldn't be infertile." In approximately 10 percent of all cases of infertility there is no reason found in either partner to account for their not conceiving. This percentage is labeled *normal infertile* by most infertility specialists. They are among the most baffling and challenging patients for the specialist. They are also perhaps the most to be sympathized with because their emotional, physical, and financial expenditure toward achieving a pregnancy is never ending.

It is important to note that normal infertile patients have no more success in achieving a spontaneous cure (pregnancy without treatment) than do couples with a known infertility problem. There is a general 5 percent spontaneous cure rate surrounding infertility which is mysterious and is often termed miraculous. It is this statistic which feeds the mythology of "miracle babies" conceived when all hope was lost. Everyone who is infertile has someone among his acquaintances who is bent on keeping the eternal hope alive with such tales. As more research is done in infertility, the spontaneous cure rate is becoming more explainable and less mysterious.

The overt or covert suggestion is often made to a normal infertile couple that the "problem is all in their heads." This suggestion may be pardoned as a sign of ignorance when it comes from lay people, but very often the suggestion is made by professionals. Physicians, nurses, and adoption workers may interpret the behavior of couples as being the *cause* instead of the *effect* of infertility. Infertile couples experience specific anxiety and despair over their childlessness. The longer they must endure tests and attempted treatments, the more evident these feelings may be. It is totally nontherapeutic to suggest to a couple that their feelings may be the reason that they cannot conceive.

It is possible that someday research will reveal a level of psychological influence over conception. It is probably true that a relaxed body and mind are more conducive to achieving a pregnancy. It is also true that women have conceived under conditions of rape, total abhorrence for sex or childbearing, and in severe psychotic states. To imply that a couple have not conceived because of something they are unconsciously or subconsciously feeling toward each other or about pregnancy is antitherapeutic. It only increases the couples' anxiety level. A therapeutic attitude and a therapeutic approach by the professional are to acknowledge the multitude of physiological components of the process of conception and the lack of knowledge of the psychological component and to assume that the couple have no willful control over their condition.

As more research is being conducted, new causes for infertility are being discovered. The physician who has performed all tests available to him and is unable to find a reason for infertility within the couple, should never send them away thinking they are *normal*. Instead, he should explain that there are many things still unknown in this field. He might encourage them to get a second opinion on their case from another specialist. At a minimum, he should ask the couple to keep in touch and to return for periodic reevaluation, as long as they wish to keep trying for a pregnancy.

MISCARRIAGE (NATURAL ABORTION) AND STILLBIRTH

It is a surprising statistic that approximately one in six pregnancies ends in miscarriage. The lay term *miscarriage* is used to differentiate from induced abortion. Approximately 75 percent of these miscarriages occur in the first trimester of pregnancy (weeks 1–12) and are a result of a "blighted pregnancy" which fails to grow and is expelled from the uterus. Twenty-five percent of miscarriages occur in the second trimester of pregnancy (weeks 12–24) and are most often caused by the inability of the growing fetus to maintain its placental attachment because of a mechanical or hormonal problem or because of a weak or "incompetent" cervix which dilates too early and allows the pregnancy to be expelled. Any fetus delivered after the arbitrary "age of viability" (usually set at 24–28 weeks) is called a *premature delivery* and not a miscarriage. A baby has a statistical chance for surviving after the age of viability. This chance improves every week the fetus is in the uterus.

Miscarriage is a very emotional event. It is usually true that the intensity of emotions is in some relation to the desire for the pregnancy, the difficulty with which the couple were able to conceive, and the duration of the pregnancy before it aborted. There seems to be a difference, for example, between a woman's losing a third-week "blighted pregnancy" and a woman's losing a fetus at 5 months because of a weak cervix. The woman for whom conception comes easily may not feel as intense a sense of loss as the woman who has conceived only after great effort.

The feelings accompanying a miscarriage vary in kind and intensity from woman to woman, situation to situation, but usually there are common themes. The woman who has lost a pregnancy feels an *acute sense of loss* and goes through a *grief* process. She may be tearful, dependent on others (particularly her own mother or other women), very depressed, and physically without energy or appetite or interest in outside activities. If she is allowed to grieve openly and honestly, and if her grief is supported by those around her, it will usually run its course to a point where she accepts the event. Complicating the very necessary feelings of grief may also be feelings of *guilt*. Both the woman and her partner may think of something they did or didn't do which might have caused the miscarriage. Women frequently blame smoking, working too hard, or poor diet habits; men sometimes feel guilty if they have had intercourse recently or haven't "taken care of their woman" as they think they should. The guilt must be acknowledged, talked out, and worked through. In the medical analysis, external factors, such as those mentioned above, are rarely if ever the reasons behind a miscarriage.

There is often another emotion: *fear*. The couple have lost control of something they achieved once. It could happen again. Some couples are reluctant to undertake another pregnancy for quite some time. Medically, it is usually permissible for a woman to resume sexual relations as soon as her cervix is closed (to prevent an ascending infection), usually within 2 to 4 weeks, and to attempt another pregnancy after she has had one or two normal menstrual cycles. The gynecologist usually advises the couple on this issue.

It is essential that a woman know why she has had a miscarriage. In a case in which the tissue has been saved and examined, the woman should ask to see the pathology report on the conceptus and ask that all terminology be explained fully to her. In a case in which miscarriage happens in uncontrolled circumstances, such as in a rest room or in a car, every effort should be made to place the expelled tissue in a clean container so that it can be examined later. The results are important for several reasons: If tests show that the woman has lost a "blighted pregnancy," she can then try to set her mind at ease, knowing that this is a random event and that her chances of having a repeat are the same odds as for any other woman. If the fetal tissue is normal, the couple can be alerted to the possibility that low hormonal levels or a weak cervix were at fault. Both of these situations can be treated. If the fetal tissue shows marked genetic abnormalities, the couple can be tested and counseled on the wisdom of having future pregnancies. Especially when more than one miscarriage has occurred, the couple need to find out all they can and be followed more closely, even from before conception, by a competent physician.

Miscarriage is especially upsetting to couples who do not conceive readily. For some reason, the rate of miscarriage for couples with fertility problems is much more frequent—some studies say as high as 40 percent. It may be supposed that the very reasons why they are infertile contribute to putting them into a "high-risk" category once they do conceive. It is imperative that they be managed by a competent specialist as "high-risk" candidates from the moment of conception. To go from the despair of endless cycles without conception to the elation and joy of finally conceiving only to come crashing down to the reality of a miscarriage is emotionally devastating. The couple need professional support and comfort as well as support from family and friends. They may even require referral for additional intervention services in order to settle their emotional reaction to the crisis and to evaluate whether or not they should try to conceive again.

Stillbirth is, fortunately, a rare occurrence. Usually, it is the result of the baby's oxygen support system failing before he can be safely born or of his lungs and heart failing to oxygenate his system after the cord is cut. Even though the couple are plunged into an acute grief crisis, it is important for them to understand what has happened, in case it has relevance to future pregnancies. It is also usually helpful in dispelling feelings of guilt for them to know that what happened was totally beyond their control or the physician's. When malpractice by physicians is suspected, legal counsel should be sought quickly and facts of the case analyzed. Nurses should be aware of the implications that the legal process holds. If there is investigation of the delivery, all professionals and staff present at the time of the birth will be called to testify and all hospital records, including nursing care the mother received, will be subpoenaed. It is essential that accurate records are kept and that nurses understanding the process and principles of testifying in court.

The body knows nothing about stillbirth. It is elaborately prepared for the close contact and physical nurturing of a baby. The breasts are engorged with milk. It is an interesting and perhaps therapeutic principle of the so-called underdeveloped countries that women who have had stillbirths frequently hire out as wet nurses to nurture babies in place of the ones they have lost. The wet nurse is an esteemed person in these cultures.

Something else to be considered when a stillbirth occurs is that the minds of all family members have been prepared for the event of a new baby. Any children at home have been prepared for a new sister or brother. A nursery may await the baby—a silent monument to its death.

Some considerations are in order for the couple who suffer a stillbirth, beginning with the moment that the death is expected or known. If the death of the baby takes place before delivery, anesthesia and delivery of the baby by the least hazardous route to the mother are desirable. The husband should be included if he is able to be supportive to the wife. The baby, once delivered, should be handled in a respectful and careful manner, especially where autopsy is indicated in order to find the cause of death. The woman should be given a single room away from the nursery area if she requests it. All personnel with patient contact should be informed that the couple have lost a baby through stillbirth. Nursing plans should include one or two consistent nurses for the woman to develop some trust in so that the normal grief process may be encouraged. The husband should be included in their talks during his visiting time. As described in Chapter 6, the principles of helping a person or family to begin grieving should be part of clinical intervention. If the woman requests privacy or has other requests specific to her style of grieving, proper arrangements should be made. The interviews will stall if the clinician uses platitudes such as, "You'll have another baby before you know it" or "Think of your wonderful child(ren) at home." These remarks point up the discomfort the clinician is having with the grief issue. The death of this particular child is being experienced by the couple, and other or potential children have no relevance to the issue at hand. Sincere concern and careful listening, coupled with skilled physical care, should be a valuable start of a healthy settlement of an extremely sad life crisis.

It is an axiom that nature strives to complete a reaction. When either miscarriage or stillbirth occurs, a reaction is stopped, abruptly, never to be completed. The grief focuses on the completion of that reaction. The couple may need to grieve extensively. Anniversaries, such as the expected due date, date of conception, date of the loss itself, are often painfully remembered for many years to come.

ALTERNATIVES AND RESOURCES FOR INFERTILE COUPLES

Too often the physicians who make the diagnosis of absolute infertility recommend an alternative, such as adoption, in the same breath. The couple should not be encouraged to turn immediately to an alternative; instead, they should be allowed a period of grief and mourning over their loss. Adoption and other alternatives to infertility carry with them problems and adjustments all their own. A couple should attempt to resolve the feelings of infertility before they embark on an alternative. Total resolution may be a long process, or even an unreal goal, for some couples, but it is important that they at least are working on it. The following case example illustrates this point:

Anne is an attractive social worker who married at the age of 24. She began to experience pain on intercourse and dysmenorrhea and sought medical attention. The diagnosis of severe endometriosis was made. Anne was put on a 6-month "pseudopregnancy" course of hormones and then informed that she and her husband should try to conceive as soon as possible. Within 3 months Anne was hospitalized and operated on for ovarian cysts of both ovaries. After another course of hormones, they again attempted to conceive and Anne developed ovarian cysts. The doctor spoke to Anne before surgery and received her permission to perform a total hysterectomy if he found irreparable damage to both ovaries. In the surgical procedure the doctor observed that both ovaries and Fallopian tubes were scarred and involved with endometriosis beyond repair. He performed a total hysterectomy. Anne was placed on Premarin 1.25 mg daily to supply her hormones and was advised to adopt a family. Anne appeared to cope cheerfully with her surgery and shortly afterward set about applying to adoption agencies for a healthy infant. She and her husband were advised that no infants were available. Anne grew angry and depressed. On the first anniversary of her hysterectomy, she attempted suicide by ingestion of barbiturates. She was hospitalized briefly and is still receiving intensive therapy.

There are no easy alternatives to infertility. Adoption, the standard alternative for childless couples of earlier decades, is no longer readily available. The fact that birth control and legalized abortion have cut down the supply of babies for adoption and that over 70 percent of single mothers now keep their babies has significantly reduced the number of children available for adoption. Most difficult to locate are healthy Caucasian infants. Infants of other races are in also short supply. Children of school age, sibling groups, and children with serious medical and emotional problems are available in limited supply to those families with the flexibility and confidence to handle them. Some couples are now searching overseas for infants to adopt. Korea, Southeast Asia, and South America currently have children of all ages for adoption, but only after lengthy and expensive paperwork. The couple who adopt usually have to be screened in a home study by a licensed adoption agency. This process may find "unfit" any couple over a certain age (over 40 for an infant, for example), who have certain medical problems (diabetes, heart disease, even obesity), who earns under a certain income, or who cannot satisfy the adoption worker that they are well-motivated or secure in their marriage. The adoption agency assumes an advocacy role for the child whom it is trying to place, but all too frequently it assumes an adversary role with the parents who want to adopt. Infertile couples may find this a very threatening situation.

Artificial insemination by donor is an alternative possible for couples in which the man is infertile and the woman is fertile. It remains highly controversial even though over 15,000 couples conceive this way annually. The couples who conceive with donor sperm usually choose to remain anonymous, feeling that it is best for the offspring to be treated as their combined genetic child. There are important philosophical and legal reasons why this is preferred. Some couples cannot consider the idea at all because of moral or religious beliefs. It is important that the couple who choose to try artificial insemination find a physician or clinic of the strongest credentials, where competent screening and anonymity of the donor are ensured. Both partners must be completely in favor or the procedure and counseling should be part of the procedure. The technique of "mixing" the donor's and the husband's sperm is no longer a practice at most reliable clinics because it perpetuates the myth that the husband's sperm will impregnate the wife or "you will never really know for sure." The couple who undertake this alternative must be thoughtfully and carefully counseled.

The childfree life is always an option open to infertile couples, although it requires a rather dramatic turnabout in direction to come to an honest acceptance of this role. The infertile couple may get so caught up in their pursuit of the pregnancy which is denied them that they fail to question if this is an adult task they really need and want to participate in. Often childbirth and parenting are seen as idealized states, offering great fulfillment and relief from a variety of problems. When the couple are told they can never bear children, they are forced to reexamine their feelings and needs in order to select an alternative. Sometimes they come to the realization that parenting is not as important as they first thought, and are able to proceed with careers and other satisfying task fulfillment, such as community and service involvement. Their identities, both as individuals and as a married couple, remain intact and fulfilled.

Community or professional resources for infertile people are still difficult to find. Aside from individual therapy or marriage counseling, an infertile couple may wander totally unsupported through the maze of diagnosis and attempted treatment, and later through the adoption process. Infertile couples are an unrecognized minority group who have not had advocacy from any quarter. If they find help at all, they are usually self-referred. RESOLVE, founded in 1973 and based in Boston, is one model of an organization which assumes advocacy for infertile people. It offers telephone counseling to provide information on good medical care and to answer questions; it distributes literature to inform people, and it supports them through group discussions. It allows people with a common concern to come together to talk out their problems with a goal of resolving the negative and unbearable feelings. This organization is a third-party agency which works closely with physicians and adoption agencies, but it maintains the confidentiality from both.

SUMMARY

This chapter discussed infertility, the patient's rights during the medical work-up for infertility, the psychological component of the diagnosis, miscarriage and stillbirth, the clinician's role in aiding the patient, and alternatives and resources for the infertile couple. The dynamics of the grief process were emphasized as one clinical intervention; case examples supplemented the information.

REFERENCES AND SUGGESTED READINGS

Behrman SJ, Kistner W (eds.), *Progress in Infertility*. Boston, Little, Brown and Company, 1968.

Kistner W, The infertile woman. *American Journal of Nursing* **73** No. 11 (1973), 1937–1943.

Klibanoff S, Klibanoff E, *Let's Talk About Adoption*. Boston, Little, Brown and Company, 1973.

Menning BE, *Infertility: Facts and Feelings*. Second Edition. Belmont, Mass., booklet published by RESOLVE, Inc. (P.O. Box 474, Belmont, Mass. 02178) 1975.

Menning BE, The infertile couple: a plea for advocacy. *Child Welfare,* **LIV** No. 6 (1975), 454–460.

Zahourek R, Jensen JS, Grieving and the loss of the newborn. *American Journal of Nursing,* **73** No. 5 (1973), 836–839.

8

alcoholism

in the community

by John A. Renner, Jr., M.D.

NEGLECT OF THE ALCOHOLIC

Despite growing awareness of the dimensions of the drinking problems in the United States, many community mental health centers have failed to respond adequately and often maintain only token programs while continuing to exclude alcoholics from needed services. This chapter will explore some of the problems mental health facilities have had working with alcoholics and will suggest an approach for community mental health centers to use in dealing with this population.

There are between 6 and 9 million alcoholics in the United States and another 30 million relatives and friends are adversely affected by their disease. Alcoholism is the third ranking public health problem in America and costs this country $20 to 25 billion in medical expenses, lost wages, and reduced productivity;[1]

Dr. Renner is Director of the Alcohol Clinic and Drug Treatment Program at Massachusetts General Hospital.

[1] "Teen Age Drinking Rising Sharply," *Amer. Med. News* (July 22, 1974), 1.

yet most health insurance policies exclude coverage for alcoholism and less than $218 million of the federal health care budget is directed toward alcoholism. To make the situation worse, the rapid increase in drinking among young Americans suggests an even greater need for alcoholism services in the future.

In view of these facts, how has the mental health system responded to this problem? Unfortunately, many mental health programs have avoided any commitment to the alcoholic. Despite a statement by the American Psychiatric Association in 1965 that alcoholism is a "disease," some mental health professionals retain the prejudicial view that this is a moral weakness and attempt to deny any responsibility for such dubious "patients." Others avoid responsibility by claiming that the alcoholic is untreatable. Nonetheless, large numbers of individuals seek help for alcohol-related problems at community mental health centers and other psychiatric facilities. In some areas, as many as 40 percent of new males admitted to hospitals have been diagnosed as alcoholics. The situation at Boston State Hospital in 1967 was not atypical. A survey done at that time showed that 28.8 percent of all males on first admission were diagnosed as alcoholic, and a total of 48.7 percent were probably alcoholics; yet in a 2500-bed hospital there were no beds set aside for specialized alcoholism treatment.[2] It is no accident that many psychiatric facilities have failed in their treatment of these patients. Aside from the failure to deliver primary alcoholism services, the diagnosis itself is often missed. This is a particularly serious issue; failure to diagnose a patient's alcoholism adequately may lead to the failure of other treatment plans since appropriate treatment for other major psychiatric illnesses may be impossible unless a related drinking problem is also under control. The sorry record of older mental health facilities must be avoided by the community mental health center. If adequate alcoholism services are not developed, community mental health centers can expect to be faced with major problems in the future.

Despite the large number of potential patients, this is one area where an effective program is not impossible, even in an era of dwindling funds, particularly if community mental health centers make use of existing paraprofessionals and community resources. The lack of an adequate treatment system for alcoholism is a real tragedy since the potential for rehabilitation for most alcoholics is good. They can benefit greatly from treatment in already existing programs (Alcoholics Anonymous, alcohol clinics, and outpatient psychiatry clinics) if appropriate mechanisms

[2] W. F. McCourt, A. F. Williams, and L. Schneider, "Incidence of Alcoholism in a State Mental Hospital Population." *Quart. J. Studies Alcoholism* **32** No. 4 (December, 1971), 1085–1088.

for case finding and referral can be developed and if existing
agencies can be encouraged to make their services available to
alcoholics. Since the majority of alcoholics are employed and already have health insurance, a self-supporting care system can be
developed once the limitations on insurance coverage are eliminated. Given the major role of Alcoholics Anonymous and its
relative lack of cost, the possibility for developing a truly effective system of caring for most alcoholics is not unrealistic.

DESIGNING SERVICES FOR
THE ALCOHOLIC

The primary focus in this chapter will be on the 95 percent
of American alcoholics who do *not* reside on skid row. Because of
the very specialized needs of skid row alcoholics, they will be discussed in the section on special problems on p. 140.

Assessment of Need

An overview of the treatment requirements of the alcoholic
reveals five primary areas of need: (1) crisis intervention and emergency medical care, (2) detoxification, (3) medical or psychiatric
inpatient care, (4) halfway houses, and (5) aftercare. In most communities, this is a fragmented system involving general hospitals,
private physicians, community mental health centers, Alcoholics
Anonymous, detoxification facilities, halfway houses, alcohol
clinics, and social welfare agencies. The patient may enter the system at any point, depending on the stage of his illness; yet he is
rarely referred to other appropriate elements of the system. Patients seen in hospital emergency rooms for lacerations may not
be referred for detoxification; Alcoholics Anonymous may not be
mentioned to a patient being treated for cirrhosis on a medical
ward; a depressed alcoholic seen at a detoxification facility may
not be sent for outpatient psychiatric treatment. Because of the
diversity of the patients' medical, psychiatric, and social needs,
it is clearly impossible for a community mental health center to
provide all the needed services. In addition, the proved effectiveness of Alcoholics Anonymous makes it inappropriate for the
community mental health center to see itself as the primary resource for the long-term treatment of most alcoholics.

In putting together a program for the alcoholic it is important to recognize that traditional mental health approaches have
rarely been successful with this population. An innovative pro-

gram is necessary and the community mental health center may find that its most useful role lies in the coordination of community services rather than in the direct delivery of care. For the majority of alcoholics, the services provided within the formal mental health system may play a secondary role to rehabilitation services provided by Alcoholics Anonymous and other community agencies. In fact, the long-term burden for the successful management of these patients may indeed fall on agencies presently outside the mental health system. The community mental health center will still have to provide services, however, for those alcoholics who do require specialized mental health care.

In relation to traditional mental health services, the treatment of the alcoholic is also unique since the role of the paraprofessional is clearly established and represents an obvious challenge to the more traditional professional treatment modalities. The community mental health system must come to terms with paraprofessional agencies and must learn to work with them if coordinated treatment programs are to be established. Alcoholics frequently seek help initially for medical or psychiatric problems; this may be the patient's only point of entry into the caregiving system. If appropriate linkages do not exist to paraprofessional aftercare facilities, opportunities for successful intervention are often lost.

Coordination

An effective treatment system can be established if appropriate links can be made between intake points (general hospital emergency wards, psychiatric crisis centers, alcohol detoxification centers, courts) and long-term treatment facilities (Alcoholics Anonymous, outpatient clinics, halfway houses). The community mental health center can play a useful role in coordinating these various activities and helping to establish the necessary links so that effective referrals can be made within the system. The most effective way to initiate this type of coordination is to establish a community council of agencies serving the alcoholic. To be effective, this council must have active participation from recovered alcoholics, community representatives, and agencies serving the alcoholic. A primary goal must be to ensure that existing medical and psychiatric facilities make their services available to the alcoholic. Regular meetings should be held to keep all agencies aware of available services, to work out coordinated referrals, and to plan to fill gaps in services.

Improved Availability of Existing Services

To make better use of existing community agencies, especially those that do not offer specialized services to the alcoholic,
there are two options that can ensure better delivery of services
to the alcoholics.

1. The community mental health center can place specially trained
   staff in other agencies (or encourage the agency to hire special staff)
   to deliver direct care to alcoholics. This will guarantee that the alcoholic will obtain better services, but it can require the hiring of
   many new staff members.
2. Alcoholism consultants can be made available to community agencies to provide educational services to their staff and to provide
   supervision for their work with alcoholics. The consultant would
   not provide direct services to alcoholics. This approach is less expensive than adding staff to deliver direct care, but it is *not* successful if the community agencies have a rapid turnover of staff.

Regardless of the adequacy of outside agencies, there will
always be some alcoholics that require the specialized services of
mental health professionals for inpatient or outpatient care. Each
community mental health center will have to decide whether
those services should be integrated into their existing units or
whether specialized units need to be developed. In any area with
a large population of alcoholics, it probably would be reasonable
to establish special alcohol units (detoxification ward, day care,
inpatient ward, and alcohol clinic). This approach may tend to
isolate the alcoholic from the general population, but it makes
it much easier to develop specialized treatment programs.

If the community mental health center decides to integrate
alcoholism services into existing units, there are two primary
options:

1. Hire staff in each unit who are especially trained and paid to work
   with alcoholics. Ex-alcoholics may be particularly effective in this
   work. Unfortunately, one cannot rely on other workers to deliver
   quality services to alcoholics. The average mental health worker
   needs constant training and supervision to deal well with this
   population.
2. Hire alcoholism consultants to train and supervise the existing staff.
   This approach is less expensive but may also be less effective, particularly in a community mental health center that relies heavily on
   staff who are in training programs. Staff turnover in such programs
   means that it is difficult to establish the consistent personnel necessary to work effectively with chronic, relapsing patients.

In some community mental health centers, the inpatient psychiatric service will also be used for the detoxification of uncomplicated alcoholic patients. Other communities have established freestanding detoxification facilities or made arrangements for treatment in general hospitals. There will always be a need for detoxification services, however, for individuals whose serious psychiatric problems make them difficult to manage in other settings. Regardless of where detoxification is carried out, it must be recognized that this is not a "treatment" for alcoholism but is only the first step in treatment. All patients must be referred either to Alcoholics Anonymous or to other aftercare programs.

Alcoholics Anonymous

Because Alcoholics Anonymous (A.A.) is the prime resource for the rehabilitation of most alcoholics, all individuals in the community mental health system should understand how A.A. works. It is a group process, and individuals are comfortable within it only if they can identify with other members.[3] Officially, A.A. is uncomfortable about labeling individual groups as having any particular social or economic orientation and will insist that the common identity of being an alcoholic is all that is necessary for an individual to fit into any A.A. group. Discussions with many people who have never been able to adjust to A.A., however, have convinced us that for some people these other elements of group identity are extremely important.

Ideally, a person should be referred to an A.A. group that is compatible with his race, social class, and employment background. In every large city, there are many A.A. groups and usually a central office that will help with referrals. A.A. is the original self-help program, where sober alcoholics, by their support and example, help the active drinker achieve sobriety. Emphasis is placed on remaining sober "one day at a time" and the alcoholic is required to acknowledge his disease and his inability to control it. Total abstinence is felt to be the only acceptable goal; this requirement is an issue that many would-be social drinkers use to justify their refusal to participate in A.A. The program consists of frequent group meetings where members describe how alcohol affected them and how they learned to control their illness. Strong support is given to members who are still struggling to achieve sobriety. A.A. is basically a middle-class organization with a strong religious/philosophic orientation. It

---

[3] M. A. Maxwell, "Alcoholics Anonymous: An Interpretation in Society, Culture and Drinking Patterns, ed. D. J. Pittman and C. R. Snyder, (New York and London: John Wiley & Sons, Inc., 1962).

has not always been a successful treatment modality for lower working-class individuals nor is it acceptable to some members of the upper middle class and upper class. Treatment alternatives for these individuals will be discussed below. As with all long-term treatment plans, it is vitally important that contact with A.A. be made prior to the patient's discharge from any inpatient setting. Ideally, they should be visited by a member of A.A. while still hospitalized.

In addition to their program for the alcoholic, A.A. has two affiliated organizations that can be extremely helpful in managing a problem drinker. *Alanon* is a group support program for the spouses or others closely involved with the alcoholic. *Alateen* provides similar services for the children of the alcoholic. Both groups are very supportive to family members and are helpful in relieving the guilt such persons often feel regarding their relative's drinking problem. Helpful guidance is given on how to respond to an active drinker in ways that will encourage rather than subvert sobriety. This program is extremely effective in many situations; relatives can be usefully referred to these groups even if the alcoholic patient refuses to go to A.A. or to obtain other help.

Halfway Houses

Halfway houses are a vital element in the rehabilitation of the severe alcoholic. When individuals no longer have any stable social situations, jobs, or homes, it is impossible to reestablish them in society without a 2- to 4-month stay in a halfway house. Most halfway houses are strongly oriented to A.A., which provides outpatient support after they leave the halfway house. For those individuals who cannot accept the A.A. approach, a halfway house should be located that does not insist on participation in A.A.

Female alcoholics present a special problem because of the lack of appropriate halfway house facilities. Referral agencies should know which halfway houses accept women and, if need be, exercise leadership for the establishment of special facilities for women, as well as other minorities.

Outpatient Psychiatric Services

Treatment for alcoholics can be provided either in a psychiatrically oriented alcohol clinic or as part of a general psychiatric clinic. These programs seem to be a better alternative for individuals who are uncomfortable with the A.A. approach. This may include both lower-class and upper-class persons.[4] Many people who perceive their problems as having psychological determinants will specifically request psychotherapy. In addition, individuals in the early stages of alcoholism may find this to be a more acceptable alternative than the requirement that they identify themselves as *alcoholics* and join A.A. This is especially true of patients who wish to reestablish a pattern of social drinking. Individuals with schizophrenia, depressions, or other psychiatric conditions requiring drug therapy can only be successfully managed within the context of a psychiatric clinic whether or not they also participate in A.A.

In many cases, evaluation will show that the patient's drinking is secondary to a rather obvious problem with the spouse or a problem involving other family members. Couples therapy or family therapy is clearly indicated in such cases. This type of situation can be best handled by an outpatient psychiatric clinic, though the alcoholic may also be referred to A.A. as an adjunct to other therapy.

Disulfiram (Antabuse®) can also be prescribed in the setting of a long-term treatment relationship. Disulfiram inhibits the enzyme acetaldehyde dehydrogenase and causes elevated blood levels of acetaldehyde when alcohol is consumed. This precipitates an extremely unpleasant reaction marked by nausea, vomiting, sweating, flushing, and a sensation of warmth on the upper part of the body.[5] Many individuals find that fear of this reaction helps them avoid drinking; in fact, a severe reaction can produce hypotension, shock, and death. Disulfiram works best within the context of a supportive home situation, where some relative can oversee the daily consumption of the drug, and as part of an organized treatment relationship with a concerned therapist who will see the patient on a regular basis. It is of no use when prescribed in a setting where the physician does not follow the patient closely or when the patient has low motivation. There are a variety of other behavioral and aversive conditioning techniques that have been utilized in alcoholism. These require the services of specially trained professionals and may not be feasible within the setting of a general psychiatric clinic.

[4] "Patient Differences Should Influence Choice of Therapy, Researchers Say," *Alcohol and Health Notes* (April, 1974), 2.

[5] E. Jacobsen and D. Martensen–Larsen, "Treatment of Alcoholism with Tetra-Ethylthiuram Disulfide," *J. Amer. Med. Assn.* **139**, No. 4 (April 2, 1949), 918–922.

PATIENT EVALUATION

Even if community mental health centers are to play a secondary role in the long-term treatment of most alcoholics, patients with serious alcohol problems will be encountered frequently. It is extremely important that community mental health center staff know how to evaluate such patients and how to determine which patients can best be treated at the community mental health center and which should be referred to A.A. or to other facilities.

The diagnosis of alcoholism is often missed because the patient does not label the problem when seeking help and does not fit the stereotype of the skid row alcoholic. Since less than 5 percent of the alcoholic population are derelicts, community mental health centers will miss the majority of individuals with alcohol-related problems unless they recognize that anyone being evaluated should be questioned about his or her alcohol consumption and the effect it has on his or her life. Extensive research over the last 30 years has failed to identify a specific personality type or psychiatric diagnosis that is unique to the alcoholic.[6] Each patient is an individual with his or her own special needs and must be evaluated on that basis. There are few common denominators among patients, except for a history of inadequate care if they have been previously labeled as alcoholic. It is important that this situation change and that the identification of an alcohol problem lead not to discrimination and exclusion from care but to the delivery of appropriate rehabilitative services.

Evaluation of the alcoholic clearly demonstrates the usefulness of the four conceptual models—the biologic, psychologic, behavioral, and social—identified in Chapter 1.[7] In 1970, only 49 percent of 80,000 physicians surveyed defined alcoholism as a medical disease. Many preferred to view it as a *behavioral problem*. In a survey done among 345 psychiatrists and 480 psychologists employed by the Veterans Administration, both groups were asked to select possible definitions of alcoholism and then to rank their answers in order of preference. More than 65 percent of both groups rejected the disease concept and preferred to characterize alcoholism as a behavior problem, symptom com-

[6] J. F. Oxford, "Personality Factors in Alcoholism: A Psychological Approach," *Update* (June 1972), 1371–1378.
[7] A. Lazare, "Hidden Conceptual Models in Clinical Psychiatry," *New England J. Med.* **288** (February 15, 1973), 345–351.

plex, or escape mechanism.[8] The conceptual models easily
resolve this conflict and permit us to appreciate the broad manifestations of this condition. This is far from an academic exercise since successful treatment is dependent on the recognition
that the patient may have problems in many areas and that a
coordinated and broad-based treatment program dealing with all
of these areas is necessary to achieve successful results.

The *medical* aspects of the patient's disease are usually fairly
obvious. Does the alcoholic metabolize alcohol in an abnormal
manner? Is detoxification the patient's immediate need? What
other health problems may occur secondary to alcoholism, and
has adequate treatment been instituted? Alcoholics may also suffer from a variety of other psychiatric conditions, such as schizophrenia or manic-depressive disease; effective management of the
alcoholism may require the psychopharmacologic treatment of
other underlying conditions. In addition, disulfiram (Antabuse®)
may be an appropriate medical tool in the treatment of some
alcoholics.

From the perspective of the *psychologic* model several questions are appropriate. What psychodynamic issues have initiated
the patient's drinking behavior and have permitted this behavior
to continue over a period of time? How will these psychodynamic
issues affect the patient's participation in treatment and does a
treatment program need to be developed in such a manner as to
compensate for the patient's particular psychological makeup?
Finally, what are the immediate psychological precipitants that
have led to the patient's request for treatment?

When viewed from the *behavioral* perspective, alcoholism
presents a unique issue. Drinking is clearly a learned behavior that
has strong reinforcing qualities because of alcohol's ability, at
least initially, to relieve anxiety and to alleviate depression. This
raises the question of whether total abstinence is necessary for
effective rehabilitation. Is is possible to help the patient develop
new coping devices and more appropriate behavior when he continues to drink and receives reinforcement from that behavior?
Often, successful treatment is dependent on our ability to supply
adequate alternative sources of gratification so that the patient
can give up his or her dependence on alcohol.

In defining the *social* aspects of the patient's problem, it is
important to recognize that serious functional impairment is
often associated with alcoholism. It is rare for a patient to have

[8]W. J. Knox, "Attitudes of Psychiatrists and Psychologists Toward
Alcoholism," *Amer. J. Psychiat.* **127**, No. 12 (June 1971), 111-115.

a significant drinking problem that has not had an adverse effect on his family or his job. These situations need to be evaluated fully; treatment often requires specific services for the family or spouse as well as adequate educational and vocational rehabilitation services for the patient. Abstinence may require a complete change in the patient's social activities.

Successful treatment requires a coordinated and comprehensive plan that is based on all four conceptual models. The evaluator of the alcoholic must also go beyond the patient's stated request for help. Patients may ask for assistance with only the most obvious medical problems, such as detoxification. Often, they are too depressed or discouraged to articulate their other less obvious needs. It is incumbent upon the care giver to explore these issues in detail with the patient.

Treatment, however, must start by meeting the patient's primary request whenever possible. Successful results depend on a program that can begin at a point that is acceptable to the patient. Care givers must be careful not to drive a patient away from treatment by pressing for complete abstinence at a time when the patient is unable to accept this as an appropriate goal. As long as the patient acknowledges that he or she has some problem and expresses a wish to deal with it in a meaningful fashion, then we should attempt to satisfy his request. Ultimately, a more comprehensive treatment plan can be negotiated with the patient, but often this will occur at a later stage when the patient is more willing to accept the major commitment to therapy and rehabilitation that is required. Failure in treatment may occur whenever treatment plans have ignored any major patient need.

TREATMENT PHILOSOPHY

Therapeutic Optimism

As in any other form of treatment, successful alcoholism therapy is dependent on the therapist's attitude toward the patient. The major ingredients of success in Alcoholics Anonymous are their willingness to accept the active alcoholic and the high degree of therapeutic optimism conveyed by A.A. members. Acceptance and optimism are necessary for successful treatment because the patient usually begins at a point where he or she feels hopeless and perceives himself or herself in a very negative fashion. Strong support is needed from the therapist if the alcoholic is to continue in treatment.

Developing Appropriate Treatment Goals

Because of their failure to develop appropriate treatment goals, many therapists become easily frustrated while working with the alcoholic and thus subvert what might otherwise be a successful treatment approach. Therapists can become demoralized because of recidivism and an allegedly high failure rate. This often produces hostility that is inappropriately directed toward the patient. If therapists can appreciate that they are dealing with a chronic relapsing illness and can learn to expect a prolonged treatment course sometimes interrupted by recurrences of drinking and if they can see control of the illness as a reasonable goal rather than total cure, then they are better able to sustain an optimistic attitude toward the patient. Thus, for each patient, appropriate and attainable goals must be developed. Evidence of improvement in relation to these goals is usually adequate to sustain the therapist, particularly if he or she is able to give up fantasies about a "cure" dependent on permanent abstinence. Other problems that present major difficulties are the depression and demoralization that can affect staff members working with difficult chronic patients. It is important that supervisors give adequate attention to these concerns and provide strong support for the staff in their difficult work, as well as provide them with congenial working circumstances and adequate in-service training to strengthen the positive elements of their job. While working with such difficult patients, it is important that the staff support each other during periods of frustration and therapeutic difficulty.

While there is some evidence to suggest that some alcoholics can return to a pattern of social drinking, it is difficult to identify these patients at the start of therapy, and therapists are advised to recommend abstinence for all alcoholics.[9] Nonetheless, patients who wish to return to a social drinking pattern should not be rejected from therapy.

Therapists must also be willing to accept a patient back in treatment at whatever time the patient presents himself. Whenever a patient returns to therapy after a relapse, the therapist is in a good position to negotiate a more realistic and often more demanding therapeutic contract.

The paraprofessional has a particularly useful role to play during the initial phases of contact with the patient. Patients are often reluctant to accept treatment recommendations at this

---

[9] E. X. Freed, "Abstinence for Alcoholics Reconsidered," *J. Alcoholism* 8, No. 3, (Autumn 1973), 106–110.

point. Recovered alcoholics often have a special facility for breaking through the defenses and denial of the resistant patient. It is important that the care giver be sympathetic and understanding of the patient's difficulty and that he persist in pointing out the problems, regardless of the patient's efforts to deny. It is equally important, however, that he avoid moralizing or being judgmental about the patient's behavior. A therapist can avoid arguments about whether or not the patient is an alcoholic without denying that the patient has problems with alcohol. Many serious alcoholics will accept this as the initial step to treatment; whereas they will avoid treatment altogether if it is demanded that they begin by accepting the diagnosis of alcoholism. Individuals with incipient drinking problems should be referred to treatment before they develop more obvious signs of alcoholism. At this early stage, however, many individuals are resistant to accepting the label of *alcoholic* and any insistance on their acceptance of the diagnosis might needlessly keep them out of treatment.

Dependency Issues

Many traditionally trained therapists have great concerns about the alcoholics' dependency and their demands for extra attention from a therapist or an agency. Successful clinics, as well as A.A., have learned that excessive dependency is the norm in the early stages of recovery and that it can be tolerated without any detrimental effects to the patient. Constructive responses to the patient's dependency needs may in fact be necessary in order to engage the patient successfully in treatment. Thus the clinic must be willing to respond with extra visits or phone calls when necessary and to reach out to the patient in times of need. One of the major reasons for the effectiveness of A.A. is their availability on a 24-hour basis and their realistic knowledge that patients with serious problems such as alcoholism cannot confine their therapeutic needs to a 9:00 A.M. to 5:00 P.M. clinic schedule. The appropriate key to managing dependency is not to reject the patient's needs during the early stages of treatment but to assist the patient in such a way that he is gradually able to become more independent and can eventually come to terms with his dependency needs.[10]

[10] S. S. Jordy, "Dependency Problems in Alcoholism Treatment," *Connecticut Review on Alcoholism* **23**, No. 1, (October 1971), 1–2.

Dealing with the Intoxicated Patient

The intoxicated patient presents another special problem. These patients may be separated into two categories. If an individual presents himself in a crisis situation requiring immediate care such as detoxification or treatment for a suicide attempt or a psychotic episode, he obviously should be treated regardless of his intoxicated condition. Such individuals should be given the same respect and deference due any patient, regardless of the circumstances.

On the other hand, if an individual being followed for long-term psychotherapy or supportive counseling appears intoxicated at the time of a regularly scheduled meeting, it is probably best that the session be canceled unless there are extenuating circumstances. The patient should be told to call back within 24 hours to schedule another appointment and that he will be seen again when he is sober. The patient should be helped to understand that it is difficult to do productive work on his problem when he is intoxicated. Experienced therapists have learned that individuals rarely remember discussions that occurred while they were intoxicated. Such discussion may provide some interesting material for the therapist, but it is rarely of any benefit to the patient. The meeting may also be counter-productive because it may reinforce the patient's drinking; the patient may learn that appearing intoxicated is a way of gaining extra attention from the staff.

IN-SERVICE TRAINING PROGRAMS

Within the community mental health system, there is an ongoing need for staff education about alcoholism, appropriate treatment modalities, and referral techniques. Opportunities should also be provided to work on the fear and prejudices that many staff members harbor toward the alcoholic. The affective elements of such education are best dealt with by small group discussions and cannot be effectively handled in the usual lecture format. Despite the fact that most professionals give lip service to the idea that alcoholics are ill and need help, there remains a deep-seated hostility toward alcoholics that leads to their exclusion from treatment services. This hostility occurs because most Americans are very distressed by alcoholics. The average American drinks for enjoyment and relaxation and can easily control his or her drinking. He does not understand why alcoholics cannot control their drinking and he assumes that since alcoholics drink more, they must be receiving more enjoyment from their drinking.[11] This tends to stir up puritanical concerns about the evils of excessive pleasure. These attitudes continue despite the fact that observation of most alcoholics reveals that they are engaged in very masochistic behavior that is pathetically unsuccessful as a way of achieving pleasure. It is important that all staff members working with alcoholics have an opportunity to work through their feelings on these issues.

Another major goal for staff training would be to help the staff to learn to identify individuals with less obvious alcohol-related problems and to give the staff the skills to deal with the resistance of poorly motivated patients. When dealing with an alcoholic, even the most minimal motivation must be identified and supported. If an individual is referred to A.A. or to some other care-giving program, linkage with that program should occur before their discharge from the mental health center. Since most individuals fail to follow through on referrals, the staff must always check to make sure the patient kept the follow-up appointment and must contact the patient if he or she failed to do so.

Each community mental health center should designate one or more staff members who will maintain adequate expertise in alcoholism so that they may serve as consultants and educators for other staff as well as for outside agencies.

WORK WITH COMMUNITY AGENCIES

Consultation Services

Despite the secondary role that the community mental health center may play in the long-term treatment of many alcoholics, it can serve this patient population in a major way through its work with other community agencies. Detoxification facilities, A.A., and A.A.-oriented halfway houses provide an extremely effective and relatively inexpensive therapeutic program for one of our major mental health problems. It is important that the community mental health center acknowledge this and recognize its obligation to support the development and growth of such in-

[11] T. F. A. Plaut, "Where We Stand," *The Williamsburg Papers: Comprehensive Community Services for Alcoholics*. Public Health Service Publication #2060 (1970).

digenous self-support systems. Paraprofessionally run programs are usually pleased to have medical and psychiatric backup for consultation and treatment of their clients. There must be appropriate staff linkages so that referrals can be made easily from the paraprofessional organizations to the community mental health centers or to community hospitals. Community mental health center staff can provide in-service training and consultation to the staff of halfway houses and detoxification centers to make them more aware of the services available within the mental health system, and also to help them develop the expertise needed to identify the alcoholic who requires specific mental health services and to learn how to make appropriate referrals of such individuals. It is important that such consultation be carried out in a spirit of partnership; in some cases, it will be necessary that the community mental health center acknowledge the secondary nature of its role in dealing with many alcoholics. If paraprofessionals and indigenous self-support systems like A.A. are dealt with in a patronizing manner, this will guarantee hostility and further separate the elements of a potentially effective treatment network. In light of the professional community's neglect of the alcoholic, acknowledged hostility for such patients, and relatively poor success rates in the past, there is little reason to justify a patronizing attitude toward the obviously successful program of A.A. Acknowledgment of our past neglect of these patients will do much to reopen the channels of communication with such paraprofessional groups.

Nonvoluntary Referrals

In dealing with community agencies, it is important to recognize that nonvoluntary referrals can also lead to successful treatment. The two major sources of such referrals are courts and industrial alcoholism programs. In both situations, the individual may enter treatment with either A.A. or an alcohol clinic, under the threat of a loss of job or a specific legal sanction. Industrial alcohol programs have reported success rates approaching 60 to 70 percent.[12] Typically, these programs more than pay for themselves because of reduced sickness, absenteeism, accidents, and turnover of personnel.[13] It is wrong to assume that

[12] "Facts on Alcoholism" (New York: National Council on Alcoholism, Inc., 1971, 1972).
[13] "Business Seen Benefiting from Alcoholism Services" *Boston Evening Globe,* November 9, 1970, p. 14.

voluntary treatment is necessary for success. As long as the care-giving agency is prepared to deal with the hostility and denial that can be expected during the initial stages of working with an involuntary patient, it can easily overcome these resistances and, by focusing on its willingness to help the individual, can guide the patient to a productive outcome. The Boston Alcohol Safety Action Project, which offered treatment as an alternative to loss of driver's license or fines for individuals convicted of driving while under the influence of liquor, resulted in a 30 percent drop in auto fatalities in the Boston area. Patients referred by this program also stayed in treatment longer than voluntary patients.[14]

Community Leadership

Finally, the community mental health center can exercise an extremely important leadership role in the community. In many cases, it can be a partner and ombudsman for the paraprofessional system and can help to legitimize the paraprofessional's role in the eyes of other agencies in the community. The community mental health center should not hesitate to solicit the support of the power structure of the community for an effective alcoholism program. The community mental health center can be an effective bridge for the consumer, the paraprofessional, and those key individuals who exercise real influence in the community.

Effective community leadership in alcoholism requires that the community mental health center be a partner with paraprofessional groups and not attempt to dominate or control them. A unified community effort is needed to develop educational programs to help the public identify the early stages of alcoholism and to develop support for the concept of responsible drinking behavior. Legislative lobbying activities are also needed in states that still rely on incarceration as a "treatment" for alcoholism. Other areas that need to be considered are the exclusion of alcoholism treatment from insurance programs and the other forms of discrimination in health care and employment. These vestiges of a punitive and moralistic approach toward the alcoholic must be eliminated if we are to continue our successful initiatives in establishing effective treatment programs.

[14] "ASAP Clients Stay in Treatment Longer," *Boston ASAP Report* **1**, No. 2 (Spring 1974), 3.

SPECIAL PROBLEMS

Polydrug Abuse

An ongoing difficulty in the management of many alcoholics is the problem of polydrug abuse. Particularly with younger patients, the custom of mixing alcohol with barbiturates, other sedatives, and marijuana is becoming widespread. Current patterns in adolescent drinking suggest that in the future alcoholism as an isolated entity may disappear and be replaced by polydrug abuse. It is important for physicians to recognize that all alcoholics have a high potential for the abuse of other sedative drugs, especially sleeping tablets and minor tranquilizers. While medications such as chlordiazepoxide and diazepam have an appropriate role in alcohol detoxification, they are inappropriate for long-term management of such patients. One rarely does an alcoholic a service by detoxifying him and then introducing him to a minor tranquilizer that can become his new drug of abuse. For patients with severe anxiety, low doses of major tranquilizers, such as trifluoperazine and thioridazine, offer effective control of symptoms and have minimal abuse potential. Antidepressants or combined antidepressants and antianxiety agents such as doxepin HC1 also may be useful for alcoholics and may be more appropriate than sedatives or minor tranquilizers. Wherever possible, an alcoholic should be handled without medication; all drugs should be withdrawn as soon as the individual can function without them. Whenever such medications are prescribed, they should be given in relatively small quantities with nonrefillable prescriptions. If an individual does require medication, it is important that he or she be seen on a weekly or biweekly basis for adequate medical management.

Violent Patients

Other patients who present occasional problems are those who become violent when intoxicated. Such individuals must be handled through firm limit-setting. Staff members must be discreet in dealing with the hostile, provocative patient and must be in touch with their own hostile feelings and be able to manage such patients without losing control themselves. Any facility that deals with a significant number of intoxicated individuals should have some security staff available to control patients who become unmanageable. In dealing with such patients, it is important to be supportive and to avoid any hostile or provocative action toward them. Such patients are best seen in larger rooms where they do not feel closed in and where it is possible for them to get out without feeling that they are being trapped by the staff person. It is equally important that the staff member have easy egress from the room should the patient become violent. In such situations, some male patients may be dealing with unconscious homosexual fears. For that reason, a nonthreatening female staff member may be more effective in dealing with such a patient than a group of threatening security men or male staff persons. If it does become necessary to subdue a violent patient, it is important that three or four staff members be assembled and that steps be taken immediately to control the patient to protect him, staff members, and other patients. Appropriate techniques are available that provide little risk to the staff and little danger of injuring the patient.

Skid Row Alcoholics

While comprising less than 5 percent of all alcoholics, these individuals are highly visible and have very specialized needs. They are rarely able to make effective use of the various forms of psychotherapy provided by most community mental health centers. To serve this population, the community mental health center must develop new resources that can provide the shelter, food, and medical care that patients require.

In dealing with the alcoholic, it must be recognized that some individuals will not respond to treatment and that domiciliary or shelter-type facilities are needed. If alcoholism is indeed a disease, then these individuals are incurables who deserve as humane and decent a standard of care as any other patient. While responsibility for providing such care may not always fall on the community mental health center, every metropolitan area needs some type of chronic hospital or public shelter to handle the chronic public inebriate and those other residents of skid row who will never be able to make a better adjustment. Facilities are needed which provide adequate shelter and meals without requiring abstinence and which have a high degree of tolerance for the life-style of the derelict. While some chronic alcoholics may be salvaged as a result of their care at such a facility, this may be the permanent alternative care system for most of these unfortunates.

Treatment for Minority Groups

If a community mental health center serves any significant minority population, it can be assumed that specialized alcoholism services may be needed for this group. Dependent on local needs and minority cultural traditions, the community mental health center will have to decide whether specialized alcoholism units are needed for each minority group or whether members of the minority group should be added to the staff of existing programs to act as outreach workers and counselors for this population. It is wrong to assume that Blacks, American Indians, or Spanish-speaking alcoholics will automatically make use of existing programs.

Adolescent Problem Drinkers

Finally, a word about the growing number of young people who are showing signs of early problem drinking. A study released in 1974 by the National Institute on Alcohol Abuse and Alcoholism placed 36 percent of high school seniors in this group. These statistics are probably low since they do not include high school dropouts who are likely to have an even higher incidence of alcohol abuse.[15] These findings can be contrasted with a national survey done in 1964 and 1965 that classified 24 to 26 percent of the population over the age of 21 as heavy drinkers.[16]

We are now seeing youngsters below the age of 20 who are presenting with full-blown DT's and other symptoms of alcoholism, the result of 6 to 8 years of chronic drinking. Special techniques are needed to deal with these individuals. Often they cannot identify with older staff members or with A.A. programs not geared to young people. Some A.A. groups for young people are now available; these young people should be referred to such groups. They may also be treated effectively in some drug treatment programs if the programs are designed to work with younger people, have more flexible treatment techniques, and have eliminated the more paramilitary aspects of some of the earlier heroin-oriented programs. An important work for the commun-

[15] "Teen Age Drinking Rising Sharply," 1.
[16] D. Cahalan, I. H. Cisin, and H. M. Crossley, "American Drinking Practices," Publications Division, (New Brunswick, N.J.: Rutgers Center of Alcohol Studies, 1969).

ity mental health center is to educate teachers and other individuals working with youth to identify adolescents with alcohol-related problems and to guide them into treatment as early as possible. It can be predicted that alcoholism will develop at an earlier age in this population and that they will present an even broader range of psychiatric, social, and economic difficulties than our current population because the developmental tasks of adolescence have been interrupted at an earlier age. The growing problem of adolescent drinking demands that community mental health centers help communities develop adequate services for this group before this problem reaches crisis proportions.

9
problems of drug abuse

by John A. Renner, Jr., M.D.

ARE DRUGS STILL A REAL PROBLEM?

Changing Patterns of Drug Abuse

After an initial period of widespread public attention, drugs have begun to recede as a major concern for our society. Although the heroin epidemic of the late 1960s has subsided, it is a myth that we are "winning the war against drug abuse." The reality is that contemporary American society is highly drug-oriented and there has been a steady increase in the number of drug abusers. Heroin abuse has changed from a raging epidemic into a slowly increasing pandemic that may again become a serious problem. There is a core of heroin abusers in most major cities, and the potential for increased abuse exists, depending on supply and demand factors and economic conditions.

More important in terms of numbers is the growing problem of alcohol abuse and the abuse of sedative–hypnotic drugs. Alcohol abuse remains our major problem and affects one out of every

Dr. Renner is Director of the Alcohol Clinic and Drug Treatment Program at Massachusetts General Hospital.

ten adults who drink. Because of the major proportions of the alcoholism problem, this mental health concern was dealt with separately in Chapter 8. In 1974, the Division of Drug Rehabilitation of the Massachusetts Department of Mental Health estimated that 2.4 percent of the total population are serious barbiturate abusers.[1] This figure is correct for both urban and rural populations and can be used by any community mental health center to make a rough estimate of the number of barbiturate abusers in its area. A recent study on a university psychiatric inpatient unit revealed that 34 percent of the patients, regardless of diagnosis, were using nonprescribed psychoactive medications.[2] Because sedatives and hypnotics are less expensive and can be more easily obtained through legitimate medical channels, they have not been associated with crime and therefore with the hysteria that has been connected with heroin abuse. With lessened public concern, medical and psychiatric facilities remain the only major agencies in our society dealing with these individuals on a consistent basis. Any urban community mental health center can anticipate that a significant percentage of its clients will be drug abusers.

The major shift in patterns of drug abuse over the last 10 years has been the increased abuse of all drugs, including alcohol and marijuana. There currently seems to be a trend away from heroin and back toward alcohol abuse, but now in combination with other sedative-hypnotic drugs. There is now less of a tendency for the individual drug abuser to stay with a given drug and more of a tendency to use combinations of drugs. It is unclear whether the abuse of hallucinogens such as LSD has really leveled off or whether the users of these drugs have become more sophisticated and are less likely to be seen in psychiatric or medical settings because of "bad trips" or other adverse reactions. The other major change in patterns of drug abuse is a steady downward drift in the age when individuals first experiment with drugs. Because of this, there is at least the possibility that the next generation of serious drug abusers will manifest even greater psychological difficulties than those of the present because of the earlier age at which they became seriously involved in drugs and the concomitant "dropping out" of society before they had accomplished many of the developmental tasks of adolescence. It is certainly clear that heavy drug abuse is incompatible with the maintenance of a normal life-style.

[1] Personal communication from Matthew Dumont, Assistant Commissioner of Mental Health, Commonwealth of Massachusetts.

[2] T. J. Crowley, D. Cheslak, S. Dilts, and R. Hart, "Drug and Alcohol Abuse Among Psychiatric Admissions," *Arch. Gen. Psychiat.* **30** (January 1974), 13.

While the debate about the relative safety of marijuana remains unresolved, millions of Americans have experimented with this drug and are now using it on a regular basis. For a small percentage of this group, chronic marijuana use will be associated with an amotivational syndrome. It is unclear whether individuals demonstrating this type of behavior will continue to use marijuana or will drift back to alcohol or to other drugs of abuse.

Community Mental Health Centers Have Neglected the Addict

The question for most urban community mental health centers is whether they will come to grips with the drug abuse problem in a straightforward manner or whether they will continue to make only a token response to this problem. While some mental health facilities have denied all responsibility for this problem or make the excuse that there is no effective treatment, others have made services available only on a minimal basis. While not directly excluding drug abusers from their services, they have failed to train staff adequately or to develop the specific programs needed for effective treatment. Drug abuse is not a hopeless condition, and it can be controlled by effective treatment. Nonetheless, addicts and hard drug abusers have very specialized needs and may not adjust well to an inpatient or outpatient program that is not designed for them. It is incumbent upon all community mental health centers to assess the dimensions of the drug abuse problem in their communities and to design programs to work with those individuals who can be best managed within the mental health system. The community mental health center should also establish relationships with the other agencies that deal with patients it cannot serve itself. It is particularly important that the community mental health center take an active role in the development of drug education and prevention programs since this is ultimately the only way to resolve this problem.

PLANNING A COMMUNITY TREATMENT SYSTEM

Assessing Local Needs

Drug abusers require a wide variety of services; the agencies capable of providing these services differ, depending on the type of drug involved. Table 9-1 lists most major services and some potential service deliverers; this is not a complete list of services

TABLE 9-1. Comprehensive Drug Treatment Services

	general hospital		community mental health center		self-help program	
	emergency ward	inpatient	outpatient	inpatient	counseling center	residential
Opiates						
Overdose	X	X				
Withdrawal	X					
Detoxification		X	X	X		
Methadone maintenance			X			
Rehabilitation			(X)[a]		X	X
Sedative–Hypnotics						
Overdose	X	X				
Withdrawal	X	X				
Detoxification		X		X		
Rehabilitation			(X)		X	X
Amphetamines						
Overdose	X	X		X		
Withdrawal				(X)		X
Paranoid reaction				X	X	
Rehabilitation			(X)			X
Miscellaneous						
"Bad trips"	X		X		X	
Flashbacks	X		X	X	X	
Allergic reaction	X					
Crisis counseling	X		X		X	

[a]( ) indicates that service may be effective for a relatively small number of addicts.

nor does it include all possible treatment agencies. It gives a graphic picture of the range of services needed, and it may be helpful in assessing the availability of services in a given community. Most urban communities will need all of these services. If the addict population is not large, most of the services listed under "General Hospitals, Inpatient" and "Community Mental Health Centers" can be provided on general medical or psychiatric wards or in outpatient psychiatric clinics; specialized detoxification wards are not indicated unless there is a large number of addicts in the community. Nonetheless, all community mental health centers and general hospitals have a moral obligation to make beds available and to train staff adequately to handle these patients. Even if all of these services are available in a community general hospital, it will still be necessary for the community mental health center to provide inpatient services. Some addicts present major behavioral and management problems or suffer from other serious psychiatric illnesses and cannot be managed on a general medical ward. Practically, this means that the inpatient services of the community mental health center must be registered with the federal government for methadone maintenance and detoxification and must have a capacity to handle uncomplicated barbiturate detoxification.

Working with Self-Help Drug Programs

As shown in Table 9-1, the role of the community mental health center in the long-term rehabilitation of most serious drug abusers is a secondary one, aside from methadone detoxification and maintenance. Outpatient psychiatric services are indicated only for individuals with relatively minor drug problems or for those with such serious psychopathology (major psychosis, manic-depressive disease, etc.) that they cannot be managed by most paraprofessional agencies. The most effective and the primary treatment for most addicts will be residential self-help programs. Community mental health centers should therefore foster the development of such indigenous self-support care systems. They should be willing to provide medical and psychiatric backup and staff consultation and training whenever possible. The community mental health center can also act as liaison between such paraprofessionally run programs and other agencies in the "straight community" that may find it extremely difficult to understand the role of these programs or their legitimate place in the treatment system. The self-help movement is very broad-based and heterogeneous. If a community mental health center wants to establish good working relationships with these programs, it is important that these differences be recognized. Many self-help programs, particularly those engaged in outreach work, drop-in counseling, and crisis intervention, are typically staffed by young persons with a middle-class background who are not ex-addicts. Some are college graduates and many have very idealistic social goals. Many of them have gone into this work because of their concern about society and their desire to change things. They may see their role in a broad, political context and may put a great

deal of effort into political organizing as a tool for drug prevention. If one is going to work well with these groups, it is important
that the professional be sensitive to their concerns and recognize
the broader social contexts in which they see treatment activities.
Many of these staff are unduly sensitive about large agencies and
professionals as being representatives of "the establishment," and
you may initially have to work hard to establish your role not as
an exploiter but as someone who is concerned and has real services to offer to people in trouble. Working with groups that put
emphasis on political activity is a new experience to many mental
health professionals and requires the careful thinking through of
one's own philosophic position on the scope of his own activities
in this area.

On the other hand, ex-addict staff members of self-help residential programs frequently have a very different background.
Most of them are more lower middle class and have come up
through treatment programs as clients. In many ways, professionals will be more comfortable with their orientation, which is
usually directed at the rehabilitation of single individuals and has
fewer political overtones. While their treatment techniques may be
very different from those of traditional psychiatry, their emphasis
on the individual and their relatively lesser degree of interest in
social and political activities is an approach that is comfortable with
most mental health professionals. They tend to be more rigid about
the use of drugs, including alcohol and marijuana, than do other
paraprofessionals who may be quite liberal about some social drug
use, though they eschew the use of opiates and barbiturates.

To survive many years on the street as a heroin addict, one is
required to have a great deal of intelligence, cunning, and manipulative skills. If there is a hierarchy on the street, the heroin addict
is clearly at the top. He or she has to be a successful crook, a successful drug dealer, and a shrewd judge of people to survive in this
milieu. Individuals who have come this route and then have gone
through successful treatment are frequently extremely bright and
capable. Mental health professionals do themselves a disservice by
not recognizing the caliber and competence of some of these ex-
addicts. If treated with genuine respect, many ex-addicts and other
paraprofessionals will be very willing to work confortably with
professionals.

Services Provided by the Community Mental Health Center

Even if your community has an effective self-help treatment system, the community mental health center can still expect to have frequent contact with drug abusers and it can provide a variety of useful services. *Coordination* of services and the establishment of appropriate linkages and referral networks between agencies are vital. Because of the usual separation between agencies delivering acute care and long-term rehabilitation programs, patients can easily become lost in the system and opportunities for effective intervention will be lost. Community mental health centers should set up regular meetings among all agencies working with drug abusers to establish liaison and to work out mechanisms of referral. Good working relationships can be easily established if the community mental health center is willing to provide *consultation* and staff education for hospitals or other agencies that may be unable to hire "drug experts" for their own staff. It is equally important that the community mental health center readily accept the transfer of addicts who develop serious psychiatric illnesses. Because of its crucial role as an intake point, it is imperative that the community mental health center develop adequate skills to evaluate addicts and to learn how to differentiate which patients will do best in psychiatric inpatient programs, methadone maintenance programs, or drug-free, self-help programs. (See next section on "Evaluation of the Drug User.") In some communities, they can provide a centralized *intake, evaluation*, and *referral service* for a network of other professional and paraprofessional agencies.

Drug Abuse Prevention Programs

Truly effective drug abuse prevention programs have yet to be developed. Poverty, discrimination, and unstable family situations all contribute to this problem. While community mental health centers cannot prevent these problems, they may be called upon to work with adolescents and young people who are at risk of becoming drug abusers. The most effective programs yet developed are those providing help to adolescents through general problem-solving and counseling services. Many of these utilize "hotlines," paraprofessional counseling, and peer-to-peer counseling. The community mental health centers should assist in the development of such services in their communities.

Community mental health centers should be warned against participating in school drug abuse education programs that utilize scare techniques or that focus on the presentation of pharmacologic information. At best, such programs are ineffective, and at worst they may actually stimulate curiosity and increase the use of drugs.[3] Values clarification programs utilizing small group discussions are the only drug abuse education programs that can be safely recommended at the present time.

Staffing a Community Mental Health Center Drug Program

If a mental health center is to provide a specific treatment program for drug abusers, it is important to pay careful attention to staffing. The most effective programs have a mix of professionals and paraprofessional staff.[4] The professionals should be available for medical backup and for supervision of the paraprofessionals. They may also do psychotherapy with patients who have progressed to the later stages in the treatment program. Paraprofessionals are most effective as intake workers and as role models during the early stages of therapy.[5] If the paraprofessionals are also ex-addicts, they should be drug free for a minimum of a year. They should also be graduates of a recognized treatment program and should be comfortable working in a professional setting. Many paraprofessionals find it difficult to adjust to a professional setting, and they should be screened carefully for problems in this area. All staff members working with addicts need considerable support because of the frustrating nature of the work. The manipulative tendencies of many of these patients necessitate regular staff meetings and strong leadership so that uniform treatment

[3] F. S. Tennant, S. C. Weaver, and C. E. Lewis, "Outcomes of Drug Education: Four Case Studies," *Pediatrics* 52, No. 2 (August 1973), 246–251.

[4] F. B. Glaser, F. Adler, A. D. Moffett, and J. C. Ball, "The Quality of Treatment for Drug Abuse, *Amer. J. Psychiat.* 131, No. 5 (May 1974), 598–601.

[5] D. Bornstein, "The Relative Value of the Medical Staff Versus Addicts in the Rehabilitation of the Drug Users in a Drug Abuse Program," *Johns Hopkins Med. J.* 129 (November 1971), 290–297.

policies can be developed and consistently applied. The most effective staff members are people who have a high tolerance for manipulative and hostile behavior and an ability to work with chronic patients without needing to see immediate results. Ongoing staff education is necessary to maintain staff morale and enthusiasm. In addition, staff members must recognize that they cannot confine their involvement to a 9:00 A.M. to 5:00 P.M. schedule on weekdays. As A.A. learned in its work with alcoholics, an effective program must make itself available to patients whenever they need support. This is a major problem, primarily in the early stages of therapy. All staff members must be willing to work occasionally at night and on weekends and at least make themselves available to patients by telephone. An effective program must be oriented to the patients' needs rather than to the convenience of the staff.

Relations with the Police

If a community mental health center plans to operate a treatment program for addicts, it is important that it establish good working relationships with the local police department, particularly with the narcotics squad. The police can be an important source of referrals into treatment. In most metropolitan areas, the narcotics officers are a highly professional group whose work focuses on the upper levels of the narcotic distribution system. They recognize that most addicts have serious emotional problems and are clearly victims of the narcotics system. In addition, most police recognize the ineffectiveness of incarceration as a treatment for addiction and are very willing to refer individuals for treatment.

Many police are unaware of the treatment process, however, and are reluctant to refer individuals unless they can be reassured about the quality of services available. It is therefore important that you keep the police informed of the operations of your program. It is equally important that they be reassured about control over the distribution of methadone or other drugs. You will find that a positive relationship with the police will prevent the harassment that has unfortunately been directed at some drug clinics and that it will also cultivate an important source of referrals for the clinic. Because of the legal problems that many addicts encounter, it will also be helpful for members of your staff to maintain good working relationships with the police to help them help your clients resolve their difficulties.

The situation in small communities is somewhat different. Here there may not be a narcotics squad, and drug arrests may be handled by other members of the police department. In this situation, it may be important that you make efforts to educate the police regarding psychological problems related to drug abuse and hopefully mitigate their excessive concern about marijuana. Drug treatment professionals should also be willing to assist state and federal authorities in the development of educational programs for local law enforcement officers. In many situations, they will be very pleased to have your participation, and this will be a good way of establishing relationships with the local police.

EVALUATION OF THE DRUG USER

The first step in the evaluation of a patient and his drug problem is to try to establish a trusting relationship. Even when dealing with a medical emergency, remember that drug abusers may be fearful of contact with the police and may be reluctant to give the correct facts. Patients need to be assured that what they tell you will be held in confidence and that their request for treatment will not lead to criminal action. Addicts have come to expect rejection and hostility from "straights;" initially, they may be very defensive and will need to be reassured of your genuine desire to help.

Assessing the Need for Medical Treatment

Before looking more closely at the drug abuser, it will be helpful to go briefly through the major categories of drugs with an emphasis on those situations requiring immediate medical attention. Patients should be questioned carefully regarding their drug use, but it is important to remember that more accurate information may be obtained by interviewing their parents or friends or by physical examination and blood and urine toxicology.

The following questions should be asked of all drug abusers:

1. What drug or drugs are being used?
2. For each drug, note
   (a) the quantity used on a daily basis.
   (b) the frequency of such use.
   (c) how long such drugs have been used.
3. Is alcohol used in combination with other sedative-hypnotic drugs?

It is sometimes necessary to check the belongings of comatose patients for evidence to identify the drugs they have ingested. Adequate evaluation of the type of drugs used is vital to developing an appropriate treatment plan.

Sedative–hyponotics. This is a large group of drugs including alcohol, barbiturates, and barbiturate-like drugs such as meprobamate and glutethimide. Minor tranquilizers such as chlordiazepoxide, diazepam, and sedatives such as flurazepam are in this group. All these drugs have a potential for physical and psychological dependence and will produce tolerance leading to increasing dosage. Acute withdrawal will produce seizures, and overdoses can cause coma and death. Overdoses and acute withdrawal from these drugs are medical emergencies and require hospitalization. It is sometimes difficult to assess whether an abuser of these drugs is physically dependent, especially since users have a tendency to *underestimate* the amount of sedative–hypnotics they are taking. As a general rule, it takes 800 mg or more a day of Seconal for more than 5 weeks to produce physiologic addiction. Equivalent doses of the other drugs in this group are listed in Table 9-2.

Marijuana is also classified as a sedative–hypnotic; it can produce moderate psychological dependence, but it has a low abuse potential since it produces neither tolerance nor physical dependence. Panic reactions sometimes occur in the naive user, but these are rare and usually can be alleviated by reassurance that the effects are drug-related and will soon end.

The *narcotic* group includes opium, heroin, morphine, meperidine, codeine, methadone, and a variety of other synthetic compounds. With the exception of codeine, all of these drugs are highly addictive and rapidly produce tolerance, physical dependence, and psychological dependence. As a general rule, an individual can become addicted to narcotics in less than a week if they are used on a daily basis and in regularly increasing dosages. Because of inadequate information regarding the quality of the drugs being used or the pattern of drug use, however, addiction to narcotics can never be fully documented unless withdrawal signs are observed or the individual is challenged with a narcotic antagonist. Heroin and methadone overdoses are life-threatening emergencies and require immediate medical care. Withdrawal states, while quite uncomfortable, are not dangerous. Methadone detoxification is the preferred method of handling withdrawal from narcotics, but some patients

TABLE 9-2. Addictive Doses of Sedative-Hypnotics[a]

trade name	generic name	dependency-producing dose (mg per day)	number of days necessary to produce dependence
Librium®	Chlordiazepoxide	300–600	60–180
Valium®	Diazepam	80–120	42
Noctec®	Chloral hydrate	2000–3000	
Equanil® Miltown®	Meprobamate	1600–2400	
Doriden®	Glutethimide	200–2000	
Seconal®	Sodium secobarbital	800–2200	35–37
Nembutal®	Sodium pentobarbital	800–2200	35–37
Sopor® Quaalude®	Methaqualone	2100–3000	21–28[b]

[a]Table adapted from G. R. Gay, D. E. Smith, D. R. Wesson and C. W. Sheppard, "A New Method of Outpatient Treatment of Barbiturate Withdrawal," *J. Psychedelic Drugs* 3, No. 2 (Spring 1971), 81.

[b]See "Methaqualone: Dangerous New Drug Fad Sweeping West?" *Connection* (December 1, 1972), 1–5.

prefer to do it without medication ("cold turkey"). For most narcotic addicts, the major issue is not detoxification alone but whether they should be placed on methadone maintenance or should enter a drug-free residential self-help program. (See next section on "Disposition and Referral.")

Central nervous system stimulants include drugs of low abuse potential, such as caffeine and nicotine, and the more dangerous cocaine and amphetamines. Some authorities question whether amphetamines are truly addictive; however, they clearly produce tolerance and psychological dependence. Methamphetamine ("speed") is frequently used intravenously, and chronic use can be very destructive both physically and psychologically. Chronic amphetamine use or acute overdoses can produce a toxic paranoid psychosis that requires hospitalization. Less intense paranoid reactions can be managed on an outpatient basis. Withdrawal from amphetamines usually causes depression and somnolence but rarely represents any physical treat to the individual or requires any specific chemical treatment. Nonetheless, such individuals may become suicidal and may require psychiatric hospitalization.

The *hallucinogenic* drugs do not produce physical dependence, but they can produce psychological dependence and mild tolerance. This group includes LSD, mescaline, and tetrahydrocannabinol (THC), the more potent active ingredient in marijuana. THC is a very unstable compound and is never available on the street. If an individual claims to have used THC, he or she probably has been using LSD or anticholinergics such as atropine or scopolamine. The major problems with these drugs are acute panic reactions ("bad trips") and flashbacks, a transient reoccurrence of part of a prior psychedelic drug experience. The management of these problems is covered in the section on "Acute Management of the Addict or Drug Abuser."

Evaluation of the Patient's Rehabilitation Needs

After adequately assessing the pattern of drug abuse and the need for immediate medical treatment, the next requirement is a thorough evaluation of the patient. With whom are you dealing? Avoid the stereotype of the hard core street "junkie." This individual may be easily recognized as a drug abuser but may represent only a small proportion of the drug abusing population. Remember that many barbiturate addicts are suburban housewives and that amphetamine abusers can be college students or truck drivers. Is the patient an experimenter who is in trouble because of a single adverse reaction to a drug used on a casual and naive basis or is this an individual who has been using drugs regularly but has not become addicted? Are you dealing with a social user of marijuana or other sedative-hypnotics who uses drugs in a social setting on weekends with his or her peers? Many young people will be brought to treatment agencies because of parental concern about such behavior. They need to be assessed carefully to determine whether or not their drug use presents significant psychopathology. Most experimenters and casual social users do not require treatment and are rarely seen at treatment centers. There is a danger, however, that they will go on to become drug dependent. Some counseling may be indicated to make them more aware of the risks (legal and otherwise) inherent in their drug use.

Rehabilitation of the serious drug abuser is a major problem and will tax the resources of any agency committed to working with this population. It is important to realize that such individuals often have multiple psychiatric problems. As with the alcoholic, there is little evidence to suggest that a specific personality type or psychiatric diagnosis is associated with addiction or serious drug abuse. Nonetheless, these individuals are usually depressed, impulsive people who, while often intelligent, have little ability to cope with the stresses of life and have found drugs to be an easy escape from their difficulties. In the real world of the drug addict, there is no distinction between the drug dealer and the addict. Do not be put off if the patient you are treating admits to dealing in drugs. In the value system of the streets, most addicts feel that it is less disreputable to deal in drugs than it is to steal, and this will often be their preferred way to support themselves and their habit. Few heroin addicts can support their habits for long without becoming involved in drug trafficking.

The notion of the nonusing drug dealer is a fantasy supported by politicians seeking to gain support for repressive drug legislation. There are indeed a few nonusing drug dealers at the very top of the distribution system. These dealers are the only ones who make any real profit from the system; yet they are almost never affected by the law, and they certainly are unlikely to ever show up in the treatment system.

A complete evaluation of the drug abuser will be greatly aided by using the conceptual models identified in Chapter 1.[6] The most immediate problem is a *biologic* assessment of the patient's condition, whether it be intoxification, overdose, or withdrawal. Idiosyncratic reactions such as "bad trips," acute anxiety reactions, or allergic phenomena can occur in any individual, not necessarily an addict or a serious drug abuser. Using the biologic model, there are two possible treatments for narcotic abuse; methadone maintenance and narcotic antagonists. (See section on "Long-Term Treatment of the Drug Abuser.") There are no comparable medical treatments for barbiturate abuse.

In evaluating the patient from the perspective of the *behavioral* model, it is important to recognize the extraordinary reinforcing capacity of the opiates and amphetamines as escapes from internal and external psychic stress. Some patients may make contact with medical or psychiatric facilities only when their drug supply has been exhausted. They may not be seeking rehabilitation, and they may be only looking for alternative sources of drugs to relieve their physical craving. Nonetheless, they present a challenging opportunity to the therapist who may be able to use this crisis to encourage them to obtain help for their problems.

[6]A. Lazare, "Hidden Conceptual Models in Clinical Psychiatry, *New England J. Med.* **288** (February 15, 1973), 345–351.

In regard to the *psychologic* model, it is clear that many of these individuals are driven to use drugs because of unconscious psychological conflicts. Addicts may request help for a drug problem without acknowledging their more basic need for psychological help. While they may indeed be motivated to change and obtain help, they may find it much easier to present their problems in terms of adverse drug reactions rather than admit to their psychological inadequacies. Even when such individuals are not motivated to change, they may be genuinely desirous of a respite from their current existence and thus present care givers with an opportunity to work on their more basic problems.

Lastly, all addicts should be evaluated from the *social* perspective. They frequently seek help only when external pressures from family, job, or court forces them to do so. These individuals may represent excellent candidates for successful treatment. Recent data suggest that such patients may do almost as well as individuals who enter clinics and community-based programs on a purely voluntary basis.[7],[8] For all patients, it is important to recognize why they have sought help at this particular point in time. This will provide effective clues for good management. Since drug abuse tends to be a chronic problem, it is inadequate to suggest that they are simply there for help with drugs; something has changed in their life situation that has led them to seek help.

A successful treatment plan must take into account all of these various perspectives regarding the patient and the particular drugs being abused. If a patient is to be successfully engaged in treatment, his most pressing request must be responded to whenever this is possible and appropriate. The crisis that has forced such patients into treatment presents an excellent opportunity to effect long-term rehabilitation.

DISPOSITION AND REFERRAL

After the immediate medical problems have been handled, where do you refer the drug abuser? Which agency or program is best for which client? In terms of long-term rehabilitation, which

[7]W. F. Wieland and J. L. Novack, "A Comparison of Criminal Justice and Non-Criminal Justice Related Patients in a Methadone Treatment Program," *Proceedings: 5th National Conference on Methadone Treatment* (March 17–19, 1973), 116–122.

[8]L. Lieberman and L. Brill, "Rational Authority," *Major Modalities in the Treatment of Drug Abuse,* ed. L. Brill and L. Lieberman, (New York: Behavioral Publications, 1972), p. 67.

client needs inpatient psychiatric care, day care, self-help residential care, psychotherapy, or methadone maintenance? These issues can be best discussed in reference to the type of drug abuse.

Drug Experimenters

If no other serious psychological problems are present, experimenters do not need to be treated; however, they should be told about the possible medical and legal consequences of drug use. Parents may need reassurance that their child is not an addict and should be referred for counseling if they appear unable to cope realistically with the situation. Parental overreaction may inadvertently reinforce a child's drug use. With some adolescents, such drug use may reflect family-oriented problems; they should then be referred for family therapy. Individuals who have come into conflict with the law because of experimentation with drugs frequently do well under supervision by the probation officer. If the evaluator has any question about the "experimenter's" potential for more problems, he can be referred to a peer counseling center or a community outreach program. An experimenter should not be referred to a psychiatrist or to an addiction treatment program unless there is evidence of serious problems.

Social Users

Social users of marijuana or individuals who occasionally combine alcohol with other sedative drugs in a social setting do not need to be referred for treatment. If these individuals show evidence of *any* significant psychological problem (other than their drug use), however, they have a potential for more serious drug abuse. They should be referred to an outpatient psychiatric clinic. If their psychological problems are not severe, they might also be referred for outpatient counseling or groups run by self-help programs. The community mental health center should be aware of the quality and appropriateness of such programs in its community.

Drug Abusers and Addicts

Most serious drug abusers require residential care and should be referred to a self-help program. These programs can be effective regardless of the type of drug being abused and work equally well with voluntary and court-referred clients. The best programs have flexible time limits, provide both encounter groups and individual counseling, and have eliminated the more paramilitary elements that were present in the original Synanon program. Look for programs that provide educational and vocational counseling to help their clients return to society. The staff should be a mix of ex-addicts and professionals, and there should be an active citizen board that supervises the program. The State Drug Abuse Authority can be helpful in identifying the best self-help programs in your area.

Unfortunately, these programs cannot be recommended for individuals with poor ego boundaries. Drug abusers who are psychotic, are manic-depressive, or have severe borderline character disorders cannot tolerate the stress of these programs. They will do better if managed by the community mental health center itself, in either inpatient or outpatient treatment. Methadone maintenance is a useful alternative for older opiate addicts with more serious character disorders. All addicts should first attempt a trial of treatment in a drug-free self-help program, however, even though this approach seems to work best with younger (under age 25) addicts or highly motivated older addicts. Narcotic antagonist programs are available in a few metropolitan communities, but they are primarily research programs and appear to be effective with a relatively small proportion of addicts. There are no comparable chemical treatments available for the abusers of barbiturates and other sedatives.

ACUTE MANAGEMENT OF THE
ADDICT OR DRUG ABUSER

Detoxification and Withdrawal States

This chapter will not deal with the medical management of patients with drug overdoses or withdrawal seizures. These are complicated medical problems and must be dealt with by trained physicians and nurses. Such patients should be referred to general hospitals for medical care. Nonetheless, it is quite feasible for any psychiatric ward to manage the detoxification of opiate addicts by providing methadone detoxification. In addition, the uncomplicated detoxification of barbiturate addicts can also be handled in this setting. Seizures are rare if the medical staff uses appropriate detoxification procedures. Opiate addicts can also be detoxified on an outpatient basis; this is not recommended for barbiturate addicts. During outpatient barbiturate detoxification, not only is there a risk of seizures but the difficulty controlling the patient's use of other barbiturates is such that it is next to impossible to know where you stand medically and it is extremely difficult to complete detoxification. Nonetheless, these problems are not so complicated or difficult that they cannot be managed in the average psychiatric ward. Every community mental health center should be prepared to handle these patients on its inpatient service.

Establishing Relations with New Patients

Regardless of whether the patient is being dealt with on an inpatient ward or in a crisis intervention unit, the basic elements of managing the drug abuser during an acute crisis are the same. Such patients are frightened and need considerable support and reassurance. If such support is not made available, they will make excessive demands for drugs. Many addicts are frightened that they will become severely ill during detoxification; they need specific reassurance that the staff understands their medical problems and is skilled in managing them. It is equally important that patients feel accepted and recognize that they are being treated with respect as people who require help and not with the prejudice and hostility that they have come to expect from medical facilities. Most patients initially present a rather defensive, hostile veneer because of their expectations that their requests will be denied and that they will be dealt with in a prejudicial manner. Once they recognize that the staff is genuinely concerned about them, this hostility will disappear. Nonetheless, many of them present severe characterological problems and they may persist in "testing behavior," where their provocative hostility is used to test the limits of the staff's concern about them. The staff must also be prepared to deal with the patient's denial of psychological problems. Such patients may present their needs as being strictly medical and deny the psychological factors underlying their addiction. The staff must learn how to confront such patients tactfully with the seriousness of their problems and their need for long-term treatment.

Treating the "Bad Trip"

These are acute anxiety and panic reactions that occasionally occur among naive LSD users who have not been adequately prepared for the physical and psychological sensations associated with psychedelic drug use. Psychedelic drugs usually produce alterations in visual and other sensory perceptions. Ordinarily, the user is quite aware that these perceptions are drug-induced. At some point during the "trip," however, the user may forget that the illusions are drug-induced or the individual may panic and become frightened that the illusions will last forever. Auditory hallucinations are rare and suggest an underlying psychotic process.

Patients on a "bad trip" should be placed in a quiet room, either with a trusted friend or with one staff member who can spend several hours to "talk them down." Techniques to be used include quiet reassurance that what they are experiencing is drug-related and will shortly disappear and that they will not incur any permanent damage from the drug. Any distortions of physical or psychological reality that are verbalized must be countered with effective reality testing. The therapist must be careful not to upset or threaten the patient; anything you do will be altered because of his or her distorted perceptions. A hostile comment can easily set off an extreme panic reaction.

Medication should not be used unless you have been unable to calm the patient by talking him or her down. Chlordiazepoxide (25 mg) or diazepam (10 mg) will calm most patients if needed. Phenothiazines (chlorpramazine, 50 mg orally) should be used only in severe cases where you can no longer communicate verbally with the patient.[9] This dose can be repeated hourly if necessary. Intramuscular medications should be avoided unless the patient's behavior is a threat to himself or to others.

Flashbacks

These are transient reoccurrences of part of a previous psychedelic drug experience. There are primarily three types. The most common is a reoccurrence of *visual distortions* and pseudo-hallucinations (intense colors, "trails," micropsia, seeing geometric forms in objects, etc.). Some individuals experience *emotional flashbacks* where they relive an intense emotional experience (panic, joy, loneliness, etc.) that had occurred during the original trip. Least common are *somatic flashbacks* consisting of feelings of pain or paresthesias. Flashbacks are more likely to occur after an initial "bad trip," especially if it was interrupted by a traumatic experi-

[9] D. E. Smith, "The Trip—There and Back," *Major Modalities in the Treatment of Drug Abuse*, ed. L. Brill and L. Lieberman (New York: Behavioral Publications, 1972), p. 267.

ence such as hospitalization rather than being treated by being "talked down."[10] Flashbacks may occur after one or any number of uses of psychedelics and have been reported occurring as long as 18 months after the last drug use. In general, they are best treated by supportive counseling and, if necessary, chlordiazepoxide or diazepam (10 mg tid), though these drugs should not be used unless absolutely necessary. Patients should be reminded that the continued use of psychedelics or other mind-altering drugs, including marijuana and alcohol, will cause a perpetuation of their flashback symptoms. If they wish the symptoms to disappear, it is absolutely mandatory that they stop all drug use. Symptoms may also occur at a time when patients are undergoing unusual stress or at the point of falling asleep. Anything that alters the usual state of ego control can cause such symptoms to develop. In general, reassurance and explanation of these phenomena will help most patients manage these experiences.

Amphetamine Psychosis

Severe paranoid reactions can occur in amphetamine abusers either after prolonged use (in high or low doses) or after a single overdose. The violent and paranoid amphetamine abuser is the only drug user who is likely to be dangerous. It is best to approach the patient in as calm and as nonthreatening a manner as possible but talking him down is rarely successful. Temporary hospitalization and treatment with phenothiazines are necessary if the toxic psychosis persists. Symptoms will usually clear completely within 48 to 72 hours.[11]

LONG-TERM TREATMENT OF
THE DRUG ABUSER

As with alcohol abuse, many individuals who become seriously involved with drugs may be most effectively treated by agencies outside the usual mental health system. Nonetheless, there are many times when such individuals will come in contact with mental health agencies or may have particular problems that require specific psychiatric management. The appropriate role of the mental health

[10]G. Schoener, "Flashbacks or Flashes," *STASH Capsules* 5, No. 4 (August 1973).

[11]D. E. Smith, "The Trip—There and Back," p. 281.

system in dealing with these individuals will be described on the basis of specific types of treatment available. When dealing with serious drug abusers or addicts, specialized techniques are necessary. The usual psychiatric approaches of hospitalization or outpatient psychotherapy are rarely of any use to this difficult patient population. Hospitalization may be needed at points of crisis, such as suicide attempts, and medical care may be needed as a result of overdoses or detoxification needs, but long-term rehabilitation can be carried out best by self-help programs.

Outpatient Psychotherapy

Individual psychotherapy may be of some use to individuals who have *completed* a paraprofessional treatment program and have had several months or a year of drug abstinence. Such people find that there are particular psychological issues that they can work on in psychotherapy that were not dealt with sufficiently in the encounter groups found in most drug rehabilitation programs. These individuals may well be appropriate patients for long-term outpatient psychotherapy.

Nonetheless, we caution against placing addicts in individual psychotherapy until they have had a fairly lengthy period during which their drug use has been under good control. Unless the psychotherapist has had intensive experience dealing with drug abusers, it is unlikely that treatment of this nature will be successful.

Group therapy may also be useful for some addicts, but this can be more easily obtained through drug counseling programs. If specialized treatments such as couples or family therapy are needed, this is an appropriate service for a community mental health center to provide. Most addicts find it difficult to gain adequate control of their drug problem, however, and any type of therapy that involves only 1 or 2 hours per week is rarely adequate to meet their needs.

Day Care

Day care may be a viable treatment modality for many addicts. This may be particularly helpful if they have other major psychiatric symptoms. If they are adolescents or individuals with characterological problems, they may find it extremely difficult to identify with the patients in the typical psychiatric day care facility and thus would not do well in such a program. On the other hand, some community mental health centers have developed day care programs specifically for drug abusers. These would be appropriate for individuals who are unwilling to enter residential facilities.

Methadone Maintenance

One program for drug abusers that can be effectively managed by the community mental health center is methadone maintenance. It must be remembered that this is useful only for heroin and opiate addicts and that it has no role in the treatment of barbiturate or polydrug abuse. Methadone maintenance treatment can be provided only under rigid federal guidelines; these limit the treatment to individuals over the age of 18 who have been addicted for more than 2 years and have a history of one failure in detoxification treatment. Many drug programs recommend that all addicts, regardless of their history, be encouraged to make a serious effort at residential, self-help treatment before they are placed on methadone maintenance. A day or two in a residential program or participation in a methadone detoxification program not followed by a realistic effort at rehabilitation should *not* be considered adequate justification to place an individual on maintenance.

There has been a major shift in thinking regarding the goals of methadone maintenance since it was first pioneered by Dole and Nyswander in 1964 at the Rockefeller Institute.[12] While this was initially perceived as a treatment that responded to permanent drug-induced changes in the nervous system, many programs have now learned that methadone maintenance can be an effective tool toward the achievement of a drug-free state. After 6 to 18 months of methadone maintenance, some addicts who have achieved a satisfactory job and social adjustment can be slowly detoxified and have a good chance of remaining drug free. Programs that can do this effectively, however, must deliver high quality rehabilitation services in addition to providing methadone. Methadone alone is rarely of any therapeutic value. An adequate methadone maintenance program should deal with a small number of

[12] V. T. Dole and N. Nyswander, "A Medical Treatment for Diacetylmorphine (Heroin) Addiction: A Clinical Trial with Methadone Hydrochloride," *J. Amer. Med. Assn.* 193, No. 8 (1965) pp. 646–650.

patients and should have a high staff–patient ratio. It is important that supportive services, counseling, and vocational and educational rehabilitation services be provided and that a program be sought that encourages a "family"-type atmosphere and whose philosophy is geared toward eventual detoxification.[13] The ideal program should have no more than 25 patients, though programs with less than 50 patients can be recommended. Unless there is a high staff–patient ratio, large programs are often ineffective and can be devices for social control rather than rehabilitation. Methadone maintenance treatment can be recommended for older addicts, for those who are less motivated and have failed in other treatments, and for those individuals with family responsibilities that prevent their participation in residential treatment programs.

This type of program can easily be sponsored by community mental health centers. This is probably the only long-term treatment program for addicts that is feasible within the mental health center setting.

SPECIAL PROBLEMS

Women in Treatment

Most drug programs have yet to develop effective treatment components for women. Many of the programs have been dominated for years by the male ex-addict and have had relatively little success with women. Current patterns of drug abuse indicate that more and more women are becoming serious drug abusers; it is incumbent upon programs to make appropriate changes so that their services can be realistically available and effective for women as well as men. Programs need to have an integrated staff with women playing effective roles in program management. Special groups should be provided for women and should be led by women. In addition, the program must be able to provide for the additional needs of women who are pregnant and for those who have dependent children. Community mental health centers should encourage residential self-help programs in their area to develop specialized programming for such women. Often, methadone maintenance is the only treatment resource available because residential programs have been unable to provide services for wo-

[13] F. B. Glaser *et al.*, "The Quality of Treatment . . .", pp. 598–601.

men with children or have demanded that they give up their children when they entered treatment. This is an unrealistic demand and programs must develop greater flexibility in dealing with this situation. By and large, most of these problems will be adequately resolved if women are hired for responsible positions in drug programs.

Chronic Treatment Failures

Much of the frustration in dealing with addicts is centered around the management of the chronic treatment failure. The natural history of addiction suggests that many individuals who have previously failed in treatment may suddenly respond to a new treatment opportunity or may spontaneously stop using drugs.[14] What combination of social, biological, or psychological factors contributes to this reversal of their previous history of failure is unknown. Nonetheless, the staff must always maintain an optimistic attitude toward patients and recognize that many addicts will eventually mature out of their illness and this present treatment encounter might be an opportunity for effective rehabilitation. The staff also must be tolerant of the chronic nature of the disease and be willing to start again with patients who have failed or previously dropped out of treatment. Such failures must not be held against the patient nor must they be used as excuses to prevent reentry into programs. Staff morale and effectiveness can best be maintained if treatment goals for each individual patient are realistic. Goals must be developed in complete cooperation with the patient and, in many situations, must represent small progressive steps rather than demands for the achievement of major personality and social changes over short periods of time. In dealing with these patients, it is important that programs set consistent limits and that they respond immediately whenever there is any indication that the patient is having difficulty. Many addicts have a strong unconscious need to manufacture recurring failures in their lives. This is usually done by setting very unreasonable goals that they are guaranteed not to achieve, and thus they continue to support their depression, low self-esteem, and sense of failure.

[14]G. E. Vaillant, "Twelve Year Follow-Up of New York Narcotic Addicts," *New England J. Med.* 275, No. 23 (December 8, 1966), 1282.

Alcoholism

Many drug programs have had increasing difficulties with alcoholism among program graduates or those who may otherwise seem to be doing well. All that these individuals have done is to switch from one drug to another, namely alcohol, and they may not be dealing effectively with their problems. Drug treatment programs, especially those using methadone, must be acutely aware of the early signs of alcohol abuse and deal with it immediately.

Program Abusers

There is some danger of addicts being involved in multiple treatment programs, particularly those utilizing methadone. Such individuals may not be interested in effective treatment but only desire to obtain extra drugs. Programs should maintain adequate liaison with other methadone programs within the community to avoid this problem. When it is clear that a patient is not seriously interested in therapy, the individual should be discharged from the program because of his or her destructive influence on other patients. Nonetheless, the door should always be open for such patients to return when they are more motivated.

Hostile Aggressive Patients

The hostile, difficult patient can be a major problem in any community mental health center but can be dealt with effectively if the staff recognizes the defensive nature of this behavior. Most of these individuals have experienced rejection from professionals in the past and are realistic in their expectations of such treatment. Once they are reassured that they will be treated with respect, they will often respond appropriately. Nonetheless, their impulsivity and demands for immediate gratification make it difficult for them to tolerate the waiting present in most medical facilities. If an adequate explanation is given for delays or if staff members go out of their way to respond as soon as possible to their requests, much of their disruptive, hostile behavior can be eliminated. Unfortunately, we are accustomed to patients who quietly accept the inconveniences and humiliating demands put on them in some medical settings, and we are not used to patients who may insist that they be given adequate care without sitting for 4 hours in a waiting room.

It is always necessary that the staff set firm limits, but they should explain why this is being done, recognizing that such limits can never be enforced unless the staff members are willing to adhere rigorously to their own obligations for reasonable service delivery. While drug abusers may be extremely difficult and frustrating, they present a real therapeutic challenge. The gratification of successful treatment of such patients is a major reward for individuals working in this field.

10
the suicidal patient

Suicide ranks eleventh as the cause of death in the United States. It is estimated that 25,000 persons commit suicide each year and that 250,000 people will attempt suicide each year. These deaths, many of which are avoidable, account for untold loss in terms of the person's unfulfilled hopes for himself as well as the profound effect on family and friends.

Mental health workers, especially nurses and physicians, are the front line defense against suicide. In order to increase the clinician's knowledge and skills in working with this problem, this chapter will discuss attitudes and facts about suicide as well as the assessment and management of the suicidal patient.

ATTITUDES AND FACTS ABOUT SUICIDAL BEHAVIOR

Attitudes

Studies have shown that most people who attempt suicide seek professional services, often with their family physician, prior to their suicide. Litman reports that 75 percent of all suicide victims had contacted a physician before their acts[1], and that a slightly smaller percentage of attempted suicide patients had been treated by their physicians within a recent time period of their attempt.[2] The significant point is that from a primary prevention standpoint it might be possible to reduce suicides by alerting physicians and nurses to the high-risk populations.

A study by Richman and Rosenhaum offers several suggestions as to why the issue of suicide is neglected:

1. People tend to treat the topic of suicide as a taboo subject.
2. Discussion of suicide increases anxiety in clinicians.
3. Clinicians may not possess the requisite skills to deal with the suicidal patient.
4. Most clinicians have not had adequate training in the assessment and management of the suicidal patient.[3]

Knowledge about Suicidal Behavior

The literature on suicidal behavior includes information regarding social, demographic, and clinical variables.

Demographic:
Lethality increases with age. For men, the suicide rate rises progressively until age 85; for women, until age 65.[4] Shneidman and Farberow found that although 64 percent of attempted suicides in Los Angeles County occurred among those under 40, 70 percent of the suicide fatalities occurred over age 40.[5]

Attempted suicide is associated with a higher risk for males although women attempt suicide three times as frequently as men.

Suicide rates are higher among those who are single; within the married population, among those who are childless.

Children less than 10 years of age may commit suicide.

[1] R. E. Litman, "Actively Suicidal Patients: Management in General Medical Practice," *Calif. Med.* **104** (1966), 168–174.

[2] J. Motto, C. Greene, "Suicide and the Medical Community," *Arch. Neurol. Psychiat.* **80** (1958), 776–781.

[3] J. Richman and M. Rosenbaum, "The Family Doctor and the Suicidal Family," *Psychiat. Med.* **1** (1970), 27–35.

[4] H. Hendin, "Suicide, *Comprehensive Textbook of Psychiatry.* Edited by A. M. Freedman and H. I. Kaplan (Baltimore: Williams and Wilkins Company, 1967), pp. 1170–1179.

[5] E. S. Shneidman and N. L. Farberow, "Statistical Comparison between Attempted and Committed Suicide," Farberow and Shneidman, *The Cry for Help.* (New York: McGraw-Hill Book Company, 1961), pp. 19–47.

Social:
Low suicidal rates are noted among communities or societies that have a warm, group succorance influence. Such groups as the Irish, Italians, and Norwegians have been cited.

Communities that are described as cold and uncaring and who do not show human concern for people in trouble often have a high suicidal rate. Examples of these communities include skid rows and other disorganized areas of a city.

Those communities demanding a strong, nondependent relationship have a high suicidal potential. In the United States, Russia, Japan, and Germany where communities place a high emphasis on an individual's performance such groups are found.

People in professions, social roles, and occupations, who have to give an extraordinary amount of concern and nurturance to others, have high suicidal rates. Physician suicide is estimated two to three times that of the general population.

Societies having internal governmental problems, periods of social unrest, or pessimistic outlooks for the future have high rates of suicide. Developing communities and groups, on the other hand, tend to have low suicidal rates since the optimism and hopes are apt to be high.

The degree of tolerance of suicide in a community or society is a factor. Strong disapproval of suicide, as an act, tends to play an important role in the individual's decision to commit suicide. The influence of the Catholic Church in the low suicide rate countries such as Italy, Spain, and Ireland support this view. Religious values do play an important part in an individual's decision about his life and his death.[6]

Clinical:
Longitudinal studies of major mental illnesses have indicated higher risk for suicide among recovering depressed and schizophrenic patients.

Prior suicidal attempts increase the risk of a subsequent attempt.

Many suicides are not reported as such.

Loss of an important person. Moss and Hamilton reviewed 50 case histories of seriously suicidal patients and found in 95 percent of the cases the patient had lost a closely related person some time in the past and in 60 percent of the cases had lost one or both parents early in life.[7]

---

[6] M. Farber, *Theory of Suicide* (New York: Funk & Wagnalls, 1968), p. 62.

[7] L. M. Moss and D. M. Hamilton, "Psychotherapy of the Suicidal Patient," Shneidman and Farberow, *Clues to Suicide.* (New York: McGraw-Hill Book Company, 1957), pp. 99–111.

Presence of a chronic illness. Patients with chronic and/or terminal illness are known to consider suicide as an alternative to a hopeless situation.

Recent major surgery. Serious surgical procedures, especially when an organ is removed or mutilative surgery is involved, may precipitate suicide attempts.

Recent childbirth. The stress of another child and the mother's inability to cope or reorganize her life may be viewed by her as a serious situation.

Alcoholism and drug abuse. The use of alcohol and drugs often causes a loosening of inhibitions and of impulse control. A stress situation combined with the use of a drug or alcohol may precipitate a suicide attempt.

Hypochondriasis. The somatic complaints of illness may be covering up an underlying depression. When the physical complaints are unattended, the person may become suicidal.

The presence of a psychosis is a serious concern. The depressed person may behave impulsively. The person may be suspicious and fearful and he may hear voices telling him to kill himself.

Terminology

In reviewing the literature on suicidal behavior, one notices many terms that may be confusing. Alex D. Pokorny,[8] in discussing a scheme for classifying suicidal behavior, points out the overlapping terms and urges an adoption of a common standardized nomenclature that would be useful for legal, clinical, and research purposes. At a committee meeting of the Conference on Suicide Prevention in the Seventies[9] a decision was reached to retain the conventional classification system of deaths as NASH (natural, accidental, suicidal, homicidal) and to refine current terms. Three broad categories of suicidal behavior (as the umbrella term) were agreed upon as follows.

Completed suicide. This includes all deaths in which a self-inflicted, willful, and life-threatening act has resulted in death.

Suicide attempt. This includes situations in which an individual has performed a seemingly life-threatening act or actual behavior with

[8] A. D. Pokorny, "A Scheme for Classifying Suicidal Behaviors," *The Prediction of Suicide.* Edited by A. T. Beck, H. L. P. Resnik, and D. J. Lettieri (Bowie, Md.: The Charles Press Publ, 1974), pp. 29–44.

[9] Committee Meeting on Nomenclature and Classification, Conference on Suicide Prevention in the Seventies, Phoenix, Ariz. January 1970.

the intent of either giving the appearance of or actually jeopardizing his life but that do not result in death.

Suicide ideas. This includes those behaviors that may be directly inferred or observed that are concerned with or move in the direction of a possible threat to a person's life. For example, taking a razor blade and holding it to one's wrist and then returning the razor to the cabinet would be classified as a suicide idea, however, cutting into the wrist with intent of committing suicide would be classified as a suicide attempt.[10]

The committee also agreed to rate each person who had been placed in one of the three categories on five other dimensions. They are

Certainty of classification. This item is rated to indicate the degree of certainty that the rater (in percent terms) believes a particular behavior is or was suicidal.

Lethality. This item indicates danger to life in a biological sense; that is, the deadliness of the suicidal act or contemplated act.

Intent to die. This item indicates the seriousness or degree of sincerity of the person in the contemplated action of ending his life. Intent may be based on circumstantial evidence such as the conditions surrounding an automobile accident. Background factors that may be considered are prolonged chronic dissatisfaction and unhappiness, repeated failures, or putting one's life in jeopardy beyond the normal course of events.

Mitigating circumstances. This item includes aspects of age, intelligence, toxicity, and organic or functional illness that might alter the awareness of the person to the consequences of his action. For example, someone heavily under the influence of alcohol might have an outburst of impulsive self-destructive action.

Method of injury. This item is used to correlate with items of lethality, intent, and mitigating circumstances.

Illustrative Case. The following case illustrates the discussed classification system.[11]

A 47-year old white male, recently widowed, cut each wrist with a razor blade. Prior to this action, he swallowed pills from a small bottle of phenobarbital. The wrist bleeding stopped and the slow-acting drug failed to cause a rapid loss of consciousness. The man washed his wounds and then dressed himself in a business suit.

[10] A. D. Pokorny, "A Scheme for Classifying Suicidal Behaviors," p. 36.
[11] Ibid., p. 43.

Main Class: Suicide attempt
Lethality: low
Intent: low
Mitigation: none
Method: (a) cut wrists
                (b) barbiturate ingestion
Certainty: 100 percent

The man then drove his automobile at a high rate of speed directly into a tree, sustaining immediately fatal injuries. He would now be classified as follows:

Main Class: Completed suicide
Lethality: high
Intent: high
Mitigation: none
Method: automobile
Certainty: 70 percent

ASSESSMENT OF SUICIDAL BEHAVIOR

A major problem confronting clinicians is how to identify the person who is a serious suicidal risk. While it is a fact that suicides will continue, no one has data at present as to the extent that suicides are being prevented. Clinicians are continually assessing patients for degrees of suicide risk. Strong emphasis is being placed on finding a reliable, quantitative measure of lethality. It is important that clinicians guard against dividing people into those who carry out a *serious act* and those who make *gestures.* Every suicide attempt is serious when realizing that a person must have few alternatives to solving his problems if he puts his life in jeopardy by a self-destructive act. The gesture and the serious attempt should be seen as points on the continuum of suicidal behavior.

Assessment of Behavior: The Nature of the Intent

A first consideration in the therapeutic approach to the person who has attempted suicide is to listen very carefully to what the person says about the suicide attempt and the nature of the intent. The intensity of the wish to die is an issue that needs to be directly discussed with the person. If a suicide attempt has already been made, this provides the opening comment by the clinician. The questions may be asked, "What did you wish would happen when you took the pills?" or "What did you think would happen when you cut your wrists?" or "How do you feel now?" or "What do you wish would happen now?" The clinician can also ask if the person has had previous depressive periods and if there have been previous attempts at suicide.

The clinician may be reluctant to ask about suicide. In our experience the patient is never hurt by direct respectful questions. The patient generally can respond to the question and understand it as part of the total interview. The patient's impulse control level and how desperate he is regarding self-destruction must be assessed promptly.

As the clinician listens to the patient describe his suicidal act, the nature of the attempt is assessed. Of course the person who attempts suicide in a severe and self-mutilating fashion is in greater danger of being successful than the person who swallows a relatively minor dose of medication or who superficially cuts his wrist. Clinicians will see people, however, who use a relatively innocuous method of self-injury with the firm conviction that he will succeed. It appears that minor attempts of suicidal behavior may also occur in psychotic or severely depressed people who lack the energy or initiative to act any more aggressively against themselves.

A second high-risk factor is the person who makes a suicidal attempt in an isolated setting. For example, the person who injests medication in front of a spouse during a family argument is not considered to be at high risk. It is important, however, that most suicidal behavior is ambivalent; although the person wishes to escape what appears to be an intolerable reality, at the same time he wishes to be discovered. Farber refers to this aspect of suicidal behavior as a "gamble with death."[12] This feature of suicidal behavior points out the manipulative aspect. Most disquieting, however, is the finding that the person who commits suicide almost invariably leaves some type of warning.[13]

[12] M. Farber, *Theory of Suicide*, p. 62.
[13] E. Stengel, *Suicide and Attempted Suicide* (London: MacGibbon and Kee, 1965).

Research is in process to devise a suicidal intent scale. The following 20-item guide, devised by Beck, Schuyler, and Herman, is currently being tested over a 5-year period to assess the intensity of suicidal intent.[14]

Suicide intent guide

1. Degree of isolation: Does the person have someone present, nearby, or no one available?
2. Timing: Is the behavior timed so that intervention is probable, not likely, or highly unlikely?
3. Precautions: Has the person taken no, some, or active precautions against discovery or intervention?
4. Action to gain help during or after attempt: Did the person contact or notify any potential helper?
5. Final acts in anticipation of death: Did the person think about or make preparations such as changes in will, giving gifts, or taking out insurance?
6. Degree of planning for suicide attempt: Was there extensive, minimal, or no preparation for the act?
7. Suicide note: Was there a note, a note but torn up, or no note?
8. Overt communication of intent before act: Was there any type of communication made to anyone prior to the act?
9. Purpose of attempt: Was the act to remove self from environment or to change or manipulate the environment?

Self-report items

10. Expectations regarding fatality of act: Did person think death was certain, possible, or unlikely?
11. Conceptions about method's lethality: Did the act exceed or equal what the person thought would be lethal, person wasn't sure what was lethal, person didn't think about lethality?
12. Seriousness of attempt: Person considered act serious attempt to end life, person was uncertain, person did not consider act serious.
13. Ambivalence toward living: Person wanted to die, did not care whether he lived or died, did not want to die.
14. Conception of reversibility: Person was certain of death even if he obtained medical attention, uncertain if he received medical attention, thought death unlikely if he received medical attention.

---

[14] Adapted from A. T. Beck, D. Schuyler, and I. Herman, "Development of Suicidal Intent Scale," *The Prediction of Suicide.* Edited by A. T. Beck, H. L. P. Resnik, and D. J. Lettieri (Bowie, Md.: Charles Press Publ., 1974), pp. 45–58.

15. Degree of premeditation: Act was contemplated more than 3 hours prior to attempt, 3 hours or less, impulsive.
16. Reaction to attempt: Person regrets he is alive, accepts both attempt and fact he is alive, sorry he made attempt.
17. Visualization of death: Person views death as life-after-death or reunion for decedents, views as never-ending sleep or darkness, not visualized or thought about.
18. Number of previous attempts: one, two, or more than three.
19. Consumption of alcohol at time of attempt: no alcohol, enough alcohol so person did not know what he was doing, enough alcohol so person had nerve to commit act.
20. Use of drugs at time of attempt: Person was under the influence of drugs so he didn't know what he was doing, drug used to free person of inhibitions so attempt could be made, drug used to potentiate the method used.

Assessment of Affect

In reviewing the clinical research studying suicidal behavior, it becomes clear that clinicians need to understand the psychodynamics, assessment, and treatment of four major affects: depression, anxiety, hostility, and hopelessness.

Depression. There are various ways to observe and report findings that confirm or dispute the affect and syndrome of depression. Specific assessment areas for this syndrome identified Zung follow:[15]

Assessment item	Interview question
Depressed mood	Do you ever feel depressed or sad?
Diurnal variation: hardest in A.M.	Is there any part of the day when you feel your best? your worst?
Crying spells	Do you feel like crying or do you ever have crying spells?
Sleep disturbance	What is your usual sleep pattern? How have you been sleeping over the past week? the past month?
Decreased appetite	Do you have an appetite or have you noticed any change in it?

[15] Adapter from W. W. K. Zung, "Index of Potential Suicide: A Rating Scale for Suicide Prevention," *The Prediction of Suicide.* Edited by Beck, Resnik, and Lettieri (Bowie, Md.: Charles Press Publ., 1974), p. 229.

Decreased libido	How is your interest in the opposite sex?
Weight loss	How does your weight compare with what it was 6 months ago?
Constipation	Have you had any trouble with constipation?
Tachycardia	Have you had times when your heart was beating faster than usual?
Fatigue	Do you tire easily?
Confusion	Do you have trouble thinking or do you ever feel confused?
Psychomotor retardation	Do you feel slowed down in the things you usually do?
Psychomotor agitation	Do you find yourself restless and unable to sit still?
Hopelessness	How hopeful do you feel about the future?
Irritability	How easily do you become irritated?
Indecisiveness	How are you at making decisions?
Personal devaluation	Do you feel useless and not wanted?
Emptiness	Do you feel life is empty for you?
Suicidal ruminations	Have you had thoughts about doing away with yourself?
Dissatisfaction	Do you still enjoy the things you used to?

The answers to the questions may be ranked: 0 (none); 1 minimum) 2 (mild); 3 (moderate); 4 (severe). The higher scoring respondents would be considered for diagnosis with depression.

Anxiety. The measurement of anxiety as a disturbance of affect may also be derived from the assessment scale used by Zung[16] to measure anxiety as a clinical entity.

Anxiousness	When did you last experience anxiety? How frequently do you feel it?

[16] Ibid., p. 230.

Fear	Have you ever felt afraid for no reason?
Panic	How easily do you become upset? Do you ever have panic spells or feel like you will?
Mental disintegration	Do you ever feel like you're going to fall apart? going to pieces?
Apprehension	Have you ever felt something terrible was going to happen?

Hostility. Based on the theoretical formulations of Sigmund Freud and Karl Abraham, it has been generally believed that suicidal behavior is a manifestation of hostility turned against the self. It is then assumed that the expression of hostility outward (toward others) would be associated with a diminuation of suicidal behavior.

Weissman and colleagues have raised serious questions about this formulation and stress the importance of observing overt hostility during the interview.[17] Their study revealed suicide attempters were hostile, complaining, and uncooperative on interview. Their findings emphasize that staff needs to be cautious in assuming the depressed patient who becomes overtly hostile is improving. To the contrary, Weissman and colleagues say that angry, complaining hostile behavior toward strangers and to staff may be indicative that the person is at risk for a suicide attempt.

Hopelessness. Maurice Farber, a well-known social psychologist in the field of suicidology, identifies the sources and characteristics of suicide both within the individual and in his social setting. Farber describes suicide as a disease of hope. He says

> It is when the life outlook is of despairing hopelessness that suicide occurs . . . when there appears to be no available path that will lead to a tolerable existence. Suicide is an act of hopelessnes, despair, and desperation.[18]

What produces the despairing hopelessness of the suicidal person? One possibility is that when competence or mastery of a situation is disrupted, hopelessness about the situation occurs.

[17] M. Weissman, K. Fox, and G. Klerman, "Hostility and Depression Associated with Suicide Attempts," *Am. J. Psychiatry* **130**, No. 4 (April 1973), p. 450.

[18] M. Farber, *Theory of Suicide*, pp. 12–26.

For example, the loss of a loved one, the loss of a body image through illness, or the loss of economic success may be viewed by the individual as a lack of competence. All these examples may be the results of a personal situation or a society pressure. Death through war, economic loss through enforced retirement, job loss, increased taxes, or illness through a socially caused condition such as air pollution could be significant issues within the larger issue of suicidal behavior.

An elderly person may see suicide as the only alternative to an intolerable situation of growing older and having to be dependent. A student may see suicide as the only alternative to loss of academic success in a society in which high emphasis is placed on academic achievement.

Some people try unsuccessfully to counteract the hopeless situation by escaping or migrating to another environment. Perhaps this is the reason that some of the more attractive and popular cities in the United States (San Francisco, Los Angeles, Miami) have high suicidal rates. People move there hoping to find fulfillment of their wishes and expectations, but they find that their original hopelessness remains.

Some clinicians believe that hopelessness is a diffused feeling state and therefore too vague to study systematically. Stotland, on the other hand, states that hopelessness is best defined as a system of cognitive schemas whose common denominator is a negative expectation about the future.[19] That is, the hopeless or pessimistic person believes or expects that nothing he does will succeed, nothing will turn out right for him, his goals are unattainable, and his worst problems will never be solved.

Assessment of the Social Matrix

Another important prognostic area lies in assessing the patient's social matrix, particularly factors that contribute to a loss of hope and increasing isolation. It is important to know the number of significant people who are involved with the patient. The greater the number of people involved, the stronger the support system the patient potentially has.

On the other hand, attempted suicide is often a sign that significant relationships are under stress, and therapeutic intervention should be directed toward resolution of the conflict. Where important relationships are highly disorganized and the

[19] E. Stotland, *The Psychology of Hope* (San Francisco: Jossey-Bass, 1969).

people concerned appear unable to cooperate, self-destructive behavior may very possibly recur.

Assessment of Current and Past History

The clinician can ask the patient to describe his current life situation in order that the number and intensity of stress factors may be evaluated. Also, family as well as personal history can be used to assess risk. A history of prior attempts is an indication of heightened suicidal risk.

The presence and nature of past psychiatric treatment is often valuable in establishing the diagnosis and in formulating an effective treatment plan. Recurrent hospitalizations are apt to occur with schizophrenia and depression. These clinical syndromes are often treated with phenothiazines (schizophrenia) and electric convulsive therapy or antidepressants (depression). If the patient is currently in therapy, impending termination or temporary absence of the therapist may provide an important clue to the meaning of the suicide attempt. The extent of prior outpatient therapy may serve as an indication of both past illness and the patient's ability to enter and gain support from a therapeutic relationship.

Aviation accidents are being investigated with a new approach called a psychosocial reconstruction inventory.[20] This approach developed by psychiatrist Robert E. Yanowitch, evaluates the key elements of an aviation accident victim's life insofar as they may be determined retrospectively. The data present a psychosocial history and any preaccident deterioration.

Yanowitch and Yanowitch emphasize the significance of multiple stresses, which accumulate in an individual's life, and which can overload the pilot's coping ability and thus indicate the potential for self-destructive behavior. From their research, they cite a case of a 52-year-old male pilot who crashes and is killed five minutes after take-off. A psychosocial investigation indicated the following stresses in his life:

1. His daughter failed in her university studies.
2. His wife was in process of divorce.
3. The Internal Revenue Service was investigating unpaid back taxes in the six figures.
4. Aircraft repair service was about to be refused due to nonpayment of past aircraft bills.
5. The bank was about to repossess his aircraft.

[20] Robert E. Yanowitch, Stanley R. Mohler, and E. A. Nichols, "Psychosocial Reconstruction Inventory: A Postdictal Instrument in Aircraft Accident Investigation," *Aerospace Medicine* **43**, No. 5 (1972), 551–554.

6. The District Attorney was about to serve him with a criminal suit arising out of an arson charge and an attempted murder charge.
7. A civil suit was being considered by an insurance company.[21]

With an extensively depleted coping ability, the pilot utilized what little coping capacity he had left in an inappropriate manner, according to the psychosocial analysis, and flew his aircraft into the ground. His mode of death was intentional suicide.

PSYCHIATRIC DIAGNOSIS

A key prognostic factor in assessing the likelihood of a person repeating suicidal behavior is the identification of underlying psychiatric illness. The most frequently encountered illnesses will be described, including depression, schizophrenia, organic brain syndrome, and certain of the personality disorders.[22]

Depressive Syndromes

This group of disorders presents a common clinical picture distinguishable from transient mood states. The patient presents a forlorn, generally immobile countenance with varying degrees of psychomotor retardation and/or agitation, diminished appetite, and almost invariably insomnia. His thought content is marked by hopelessness, guilt, anger, desperation, loneliness, and feelings of worthlessness. Concomitant suicidal ideas may emerge as he feels that he deserves to be dead, that others would be better off in his absence, or that suicide is the only escape from what appears to be an intolerable situation. Further progression of the syndrome may be accompanied by evidence of delusion and hallucinations and occasionally an associated confusional picture and impairment of intellectual functioning.

Diagnosis is made by clinical observation and direct questioning of the patient and relatives. Often he has a history of previous depressive episodes that may have responded to antidepressant medication or electroconvulsive therapy and that may have

---

[21] Robert E. Yanowitch and E. A. Yanowitch, "Emotional Factors in Unsafe Flight," Flight Instructors' Safety Report, AOPA Air Safety Foundation, Flight Instructor Dept., Bethesda, Md., 1, No. 3 (July 1975), 1–2.

[22] The rest of this section is based in part on "Management of the Attempted Suicide Patient: Indications for Psychiatric Hospitalization," by Owen S. Surman and Aaron Lazare, in *Medical Insight* (July 1972), pp. 14–21. Copyright by Insight Publishing Co., Inc, and used with permission.

required hospitalization. The organic brain syndromes can generally be ruled out through the history and through tests.

Depression is the pneumonia of psychiatry; if left untreated it often has high morbidity and mortality. Treatment on the other hand, often leads to complete remission. Attempted suicide in a depressed patient calls for rapid, definitive treatment by psychotherapy, antidepressant medication, and/or electroconvulsive treatment. When the depressive symptoms are severe with marked alteration in normal life-style functions or pronounced feelings of hopelessness and guilt, outpatient management is accompanied by significant risk. The patient may be so convinced of his hopelessness that he is unable to cooperate in an outpatient program; his antidepressant medication may present the temptation of lethal overdose; and there is often a considerable time lag before treatment takes effect. It is advisable to hospitalize the depressed patient who has attempted suicide when his depressive symptoms are severe, when he is out of contact with reality, or when he presents continuing suicidal ideation.

The Schizophrenic Syndromes

These are characterized by impairment of the capacity to distinguish reality from fantasy with a progressive tendency toward disordered communication, altered emotional responsiveness, and social isolation. The syndrome's onset may be insidious or sudden. Classically, the patient's presentation is marked by bizarreness in dress, deportment, and speech with an air of cold indifference and/or inappropriate outbursts of anger, sadness, or mirth. The stream of talk is generally loosely connected and its content marked by bizarre somatic preoccupations, ideas of a grandiose or paranoid nature, fear of thought control, and/or feelings of estrangement and depersonalization. Suicidal thinking may relate to any or all of these thoughts. With progressive decompensation these are frank delusions and hallucinations; suicidal behavior at this point may relate to the delusional system or be dictated by a hallucinated voice.

Diagnosis is made in the same way as in the depressive syndromes by clinical observation, direct questioning, and a review of the past psychiatric history. There may also be a family history of similar illness.

Although schizophrenia is frequently managed successfully on an outpatient basis with a combination of phenothiazines and psychotherapy, the schizophrenic patient who has attempted suicide is an extreme risk even when the attempt appears to be a minor one. Because of the patient's impaired cognitive function and tendency toward isolation and disordered communication, suicidal behavior is highly unpredictable.[23] For this reason, hospitalization is almost always indicated.

Organic Brain Syndromes

These are psychotic reactions of organic etiology that may be reversible (acute brain syndrome) or irreversible (chronic brain syndrome). The nature of the dysfunction may be toxic metabolic, traumatic, hemorrhagic, vascular, or infectious. Attempted suicide may occur in any of the organic psychoses but is most common in the presence of drug and alcohol abuse and more recently in the toxic psychoses induced by hallucinogenic drugs.

The patient with an organic brain syndrome generally appears confused and perplexed. Wide mood swings are a classical finding. His speech may be highly disorganized; his attention, grasp, and memory may be impaired; he is usually disoriented and frequently has illusions, delusions, and hallucinations. Suicidal behavior tends to result from the combination of confusion, disorientation, and delusional thinking. In alcohol-related syndromes, the depressant effects of alcohol are an additional factor.

Diagnosis is made through history, physical examination, and laboratory tests.

Like all persons in psychotic states, these patients are highly unpredictable and require close observation following a suicide attempt. Once medical management has successfully reversed central nervous system impairment, it is necessary to perform a careful psychological reassessment, particularly when the etiology is related to drug or alcohol abuse. The disturbed patient with limited adaptive resources whose history is characterized by impulsive behavior and who deals with stress by resorting to some form of intoxication is likely to repeat the patterns, which results in central nervous system impairment and suicidal behavior. In such cases, psychiatric hospitalization is often advisable.

Personality Disorders

These consist of a broad group of characterological impairments. Patients who have attempted suicide frequently present

[23] E. S. Shneidman and D. M. Lane, "Psychologic and Social Work Clues to Suicide in a Schizophrenic," Shneidman and Farberow, *Clues to Suicide.* (London: Mac Gibbon and Kee, 1957) pp. 170–187.

life-styles characteristic of three major subgroups: hysterical personality, antisocial personality, and chronic alcoholism.[24]

Although hysterical personality does occur in both sexes, the classic hysteric is young, female, and coquettish and is inclined to histrionic behavior. Attempted suicide in these patients is often a dramatic display or the acting out of an interpersonal conflict. Their demanding dependency frequently antagonizes others (especially the medical staff) and evokes an angry response; a power struggle may then ensue in which the patient becomes increasingly willful and intransigent. This is best avoided if one views the suicide attempt objectively, as an immature and maladaptive means of dealing with life stress. The major goal in management is to support the patient through the crisis and encourage more healthy and socially appropriate modes of problem solving. This is best initiated by mobilizing support from family and friends and by referral to a mental health professional. Although these patients require a great deal of help and careful follow-up, hospitalization can most often be avoided.

The patient with an antisocial personality is characteristically impulsive, demanding, manipulative, and egocentric and has a history of behavior that is injurious to others. Like the hysteric, he is often highly engaging in the absence of stress but meets frustration with frantic attempts to manipulate the social situation. The suicide attempt is often such a desperate maneuver. The patient needs support to get through the crisis, but one frequently encounters the difficulty that these patients often present highly unrealistic demands. Again there is a risk that anger on the part of the clinician will cause increasingly willful behavior. Management therefore requires both support and firm limit-setting as the clinician offers his assistance while clearly defining the reality of the situation and the patient's responsibility. If this approach fails and the patient is unable to cooperate, hospitalization is often advisable.

The alcoholic also often exhibits demanding, dependent behavior and disordered interpersonal relationships. The major problem in dealing with him is that ongoing stress often leads to increased alcohol consumption, and intoxication in turn leads to depression and overwhelms the patient's capacity for adaptive behavior leaving him vulnerable to impulsive and self-destructive behavior. It is generally best to encourage withdrawal in a hospital setting. Following withdrawal, the alcoholic must have therapeutic supports that will meet some of his dependency needs and at the same time assistance in developing realistic means of

[24] E. Stengel, *Suicide and Attempted Suicide.*

dealing with stress. Anger on the part of the physician increases the alcoholic's belief that the world is hostile and leads to further disorganization and self-destructive behavior.

MANAGEMENT OF SUICIDAL BEHAVIOR

The suicide crisis is a common psychiatric emergency that is seen in outpatient settings such as in emergency departments of general hospitals. Since there is an ever-present danger that the suicide attempt will be repeated with lethal consequences, psychiatric consultation is advisable. When such consultation is not available, the most important decision following treatment for the crisis is whether to hospitalize the person in a psychiatric facility or refer him for outpatient evaluation.

Patient's attitude about the attempt. Where there is no sign of psychosis, severe depression, or a highly disordered personality structure and where the social situation is relatively stable and the attempt has not been of a highly lethal nature, one can be further reassured if the patient regrets his recent suicidal behavior and ensures that he will return for help if future events threaten to overwhelm him. Alternatively, one should never disregard a patient who states that he is sorry he did not succeed or threatens to try again. Such an individual is clearly asking for help, however disordered the nature of his communication. One should also be extremely cautious about the patient who has suffered a loss and believes that death will reunite him with a loved one.

Just as the suicide act communicates a wish for escape and at the same time a plea for rescue so the wish for rescue is frequently associated with a tendency to alienate the helper. The suicide act is often an expression of the patient's rage against the environment turned in against himself,[25] what Shneidman has called "murder in the 180th degree."[26] This is of consequence in management because the patient's anger and hopelessness may evoke similar feelings from even the most empathetic clinician and increase the patient's tendency to see his environment as hostile and unforgiving.

[25] S. Freud, "Mourning and Melancholia," in *The Standard Edition of the Complete Psychological Works of Sigmund Freud*, Vol. 14. (London: Hogarth Press, 1957), pp. 243–258.

[26] E. S. Shneidman, *On the Nature of Suicide* (San Francisco: Jossey-Bass, 1969), pp. 1–30.

During the initial interview it is essential to listen very carefully to what the person says about the nature of the suicidal intent. Following this assessment, it is important to assess his feelings of inadequacy in coping with the immediate and chronic stresses in his life, his level of hope, and his view of the situation as being intolerable. The clinician listens and tries to understand the patient's view of his existence at that very moment.

In our experience, people who make suicide attempts are out of a caring system. That is, they are not being cared for by a professional or mental health worker. People who are successful in their suicidal behavior are generally not actively engaged in treatment. They may be involved in situations where the therapist has terminated or is on vacation or is in the process of leaving and thus the patient is in transit.

The main intervention in this type of situation is that someone takes responsibility to care and to watch over the patient. A danger for clinicians is to be kept so busy making referrals for the suicidal person that in essence he receives no care. We caution against this danger of making transfers and referrals, which gives the message that no one in the system really cares. The quality of hopelessness decreases when the patient feels someone does care in a human way. When the patient feels this, he believes there is some hope and this feeling may be a lifeline at that point in time.

Inpatient Hospitalization

The risk of repeated suicidal behavior and the indications for hospitalization can be assessed with reference to the psychiatric diagnosis, nature of intent, social matrix, and current and past history. Hospitalization is indicated when there is high risk in any of these areas.

Inpatient psychiatric units of hospitals are a major resource for referral of the suicidal person. These units have a dual task. On one hand, they have an administrative obligation to prevent suicide and to protect the patient by removing harmful objects such as razor blades and extra medicines. They also provide the caring aspect of the therapeutic environment.

Innovative Interventions

An alternative to hospitalization has been to test various resources that might be used for treatment of the suicidal patient. We discuss two that may be used in conjunction with psychotherapy as well as for inpatient or outpatient settings.

Patient monitoring. A clinical method proposed by Robert C. Drye[27] and colleagues is to share the evaluation task with the patient. The rationale is that the patient is the one who is making the decision whether to kill himself or not and that he has the best data as to how intense his urge is and how strong his controls are. The evaluator has the patient state how long and under what conditions he trusts himself to stay alive and exercise control over his impulses. This approach is suggested in any setting as well as over the telephone, although there the evaluator will not have the visual data available to him.

This method is used whenever suicide ideation is suspected. Drye and colleagues suspect suicidal fantasies in any depressed person and in many patients with heart problems and other life-threatening illnesses. They always investigate inappropriate laughter that occurs during discussions of bad predictions such as illness, business failure, and divorce. A question frequently asked by the clinician relates to important predictions people make, often out of awareness. Questions such as "If things go badly for you, what will your life be like a year from now?" All suicidal and self-destructive fantasies are carefully explored with the person such as accidents; abuse of food, alcohol, or drugs; or exhausting work habits.

When the suicidal fantasies are verbalized, the interviewer asks the person to make the following statement: "No matter what happens, I will not kill myself, accidently or on purpose, at any time" and to report his internal response to the statement. The evaluator dismisses suicide as a management concern if the person reports a feeling of confidence in the statement, with no direct or indirect qualifications and with no incongruous voice tones or body motions. It is noted that patients will frequently experience relief after making the statement. This intervention helps to settle the suicidal fantasy that may have been used as a delaying tactic in dealing with other reality or interpersonal or intrapsychic problems.

The person for whom suicide is an important issue either will object to or will qualify the statement by saying, "I can't" or "I won't." The person who cannot make the statement is assumed to be suicidal. He is then advised that it is to be his choice to make the statement with whatever qualifications he wishes or he can have the staff make other arrangements for his safety. If the person says, "I can't," the evaluator asks him to say, "I won't" and

---

[27] R. C. Drye, R. L. Goulding, and M. E. Goulding, "No-Suicide Decisions: Patient Monitoring of Suicidal Risk," *Am. J. Psychiatry* 130, No. 2 (February 1973), p. 172.

to report if that brings him any closer to what he is actually feeling. With this data, the evaluator can classify the person as representing no risk, a very high risk, or a qualified risk.

The giving up of a suicidal fantasy may be psychodynamically understood as a loss of a problem-solving technique as well as a fantasy gratification. Qualifications enable the person to avoid the loss psychologically since the person retains his basic position of "I will stay alive if" and has not made the decision not to kill himself. There are three qualifications identified by Drye and colleagues:

1. *Until.* Time is the easiest qualification. The person is asked to state the longest period he can agree to. For example, a 1-hour period allows the person to make short moves unescorted such as to a therapist's office setting or to the hospital inpatient unit. A 6-month period offers time for detailed psychotherapeutic work. All decisions are renewed before their time expiration.

2. *I will not kill myself.* The key words are the first two words. The decision made by the person is not an agreement with the clinician but a self-contained choice. If the person says "Nothing will happen" or "I won't try anything" or "I'd like to," all are answered by the clinician with "But will you?" The patient statement of "I promise" is considered a shaky statement.

3. *No matter what.* This qualification enables the person to shift the suicide act to someone else or something else. Common statements: "Unless I get upset (tired, drunk); unless school or work gets better." The goal of this qualification is to get the person past these external sources of trouble.

This combined diagnosis and intervention technique is reported to have a high degree of effectiveness in decreasing patient and staff anxiety. It is recommended as suitable for inexperienced nonprofessionals as well as experienced professionals. This method is not recommended for patients with organic impairment, those who use alcohol or other drugs heavily, and others who have made suicide the central theme of their lives.

Videotape confrontation. A new treatment approach in mental health practice in the emergency department is the use of videotape. This technique was tried with suicide attempters as part of a suicide research project. Resnik and colleagues[28] report that this method challenges the patient denial of despair and suicide intent by confronting him with the consequences of his suicidal behavior. When a person is brought into the emergency

[28] H. L. P. Resnik et al., "Videotape Confrontation After Attempted Suicide," *Am. J. Psychiatry* **130**, No. 4 (April 1973), p. 460–63.

ward following a suicidal attempt, consent for videotaping is obtained from the patient or a relative. The patient's condition, the lifesaving measures taken, and the interaction with the hospital staff are recorded. The patient is then transferred to intensive care, surgery, or the psychiatric inpatient service. After two individual therapy sessions he is taken to a videotape session, in which his emergency room behavior is viewed. The goal of showing the 10-minute segment is to engage the person in psychotherapy.

The use of videotape confrontation very often breaks through the defensive structure of patients and allows them to feel the feelings of desperation or hopelessness. It is noted that frequently patients will vent their hostility upon the therapist as being their predominantly initial defensive position. This focus often aids in stimulating further interaction on a feeling level with the goal of the patients being for them to understand some of the issues leading to the suicidal behavior and for them to assume responsibility for their behavior.

This type of intervention will be studied for use with families who reinforce the patient's denial, who refuse to become involved, and who insist that the attempt was accidental. This intervention is also being evaluated for use with patients engaged in self-destructive acts such as the epileptic who is difficult to manage or the juvenile diabetic who is continually brought into the emergency ward in a coma as the result of neglecting to take medication.

SUMMARY

Suicide is a complicated and disquieting part of human history. The increase of the act of suicide in our society is of serious concern to the mental health profession, social scientists, and the general public. Suicide, unlike other reasons for death, is avoidable in many situations. A voluntary death must be viewed as a loss to the victim's personal associates as well as a loss to the society in terms of the individual's worth and contribution.

This chapter has examined some of the attitudes and facts about suicidal behavior and has presented a detailed assessment of suicidal behavior in terms of nature of the intent, affect on the patient, the social matrix, and current and past history.

Hospitalization is indicated when positive high-risk findings occur in any of these areas:

Psychiatric diagnosis: When the patient has severe depression, schizophrenia, organic brain disease, or those types of personality disorders where the patient is highly impulsive, lacking in judgment, and unable to cooperate.

Social matrix: When age, sex, occurrence of loss, and the nature of interpersonal relationships suggest a high degree of hopelessness and social isolation.

Nature of the attempt: When the agent and setting of the attempt are of a highly lethal nature and have little provision for rescue.

The patient's attitude about the attempt: When the patient directly or indirectly threatens repeated suicidal behavior.

Past history: When the composite picture provided by the family history, past suicidal behavior, and history of psychiatric treatment is of a malignant nature.

11
victims of violence

With the increase of violence and aggression in our society, a new area of study is developing in the field of victimology in an attempt to identify and understand victim reaction to crime. Few categories of human behavior provoke more gut level response than that of violence. Until recently, the literature was substantially focused on the offender with little being written about the victims and their families' reaction to the crime. This chapter is an attempt to correct this situation.

Currently, society is becoming more aware of this inequity and is paying more attention to the effect of violence on the victim and family. Newspaper articles are attempting to bring the problem to the people as evidenced in one paper.

> . . . their names appear in police reports, in newspapers, are heard on the air . . . and then forgotten. They are the victims of crimes of violence—people nobody seem to care about.[1]

[1] Bob Hassett, "Shooting Left Him a Paraplegic," *Boston Herald American*, June 4, 1974.

Clinicians are in a key position to counsel victims of violence because of their close association with facilities where victims come for help—the emergency wards, community health centers, and mental health facilities. Although there is a limited amount of research available on the subject, we would like to present some reported cases of violence along with our own work with victims and their families. We hope this material will increase clinicians' awareness of the problem and hopefully encourage them to become involved in the study of trauma reactions to victim situations.

A TYPOLOGY OF ATTACK

In a study of rape victims, a typology was devised in terms of how the assailant gained access to his victim; that is, his style of attack.[2] It was noted that the style of attack was an important aspect of the victim's reaction and recovery progress. Two main styles were identified: the blitz and the confidence.

The "mark," to use the language of the criminal world, is the person designed to become a victim of some form of illegal exploitation. It appears that victims are set up as marks in two ways: They are either singled out for a sudden surprise attack or they are deliberately deceived and betrayed in an attack that has the qualities of the confidence game. This typology of attack can be applied to cases of murder, attempted murder, rape, and kidnapping.

The Blitz Attack

The blitz attack occurs suddenly and without prior interaction of any kind between assailant and victim. A person is leading a normal everyday life. A split second later that life-style is disrupted and that individual is a victim. From the victim's point of view, there is no ready explanation for the assailant's presence. In the attack, the assailant suddenly appears, his presence is inappropriate, he is uninvited, and he forces himself into the situation. Often he selects an anonymous victim and tries to remain anonymous himself. He may wear a mask or gloves or cover the victim's face as he attacks.

[2] A. W. Burgess and L. L. Holmstrom, *Rape: Victims of Crisis* (Bowie, Md.: R. J. Brady Company, 1974).

Murder. The following case reported in the newspaper is a common example of a murder in which there are no suspects and no apparent reason why the victim was selected.[3]

> Nobody knows the reason the man died at age 38. They only know the way he died . . . . A bullet from a high-powered rifle hit him in the head as he walked toward his car at the end of the work day to drive . . . to his wife and four children . . . . The violence that he hated so much struck him down in the parking lot . . . where he was employed as an engineer.

In attempting to find a reason, the police said they had no clues or ideas as to why the man was murdered. His widow had this to say:

> It might have been a case of mistaken identify . . . . I will never believe it was meant for him. There was no reason it should be meant for him. We never did anything to be ashamed of.

Rape. In the following case, which was referred to the Boston Victim Counseling Program, three young women were robbed and raped in a blitz attack in the early hours of the morning by three men who crawled into their apartment through a first-floor window. The three women were asleep in separate rooms when the assailants entered. The women were tied with electrical cord and gagged. The attacks were carried out in darkness with each man selecting his victim. The assailants moved around the apartment by lighting matches. One of the victims recounts the experience as follows:

> I woke to hear Janie screaming and thought she was having a nightmare so I went into the room to check on her. That is when I discovered the men with their hands around her neck. I tried to say no one else was in the apartment but one of the men said he knew there were three of us . . . . One of the men then got the third roommate and tied us all together—bound our wrists, put tape on our mouths, and blindfolded us. Then I think they searched the apartment and took things in and out—there must have been a car outside . . . . Then each one of them took one of us into a bedroom and raped us . . . . The men cut the telephone wires . . . . After they had left, we untied ourselves and went next door and had the neighbor call the police.

[3] Bob Hassett, "Widows Ready to Join 'People vs. Handguns'," *Boston Herald American*, June 6, 1974.

All three women thought they would be killed, and as one victim said:

> I kept telling myself to stay calm—I can get hysterical. We are lucky to be alive—I thought we would be killed.

Murder and attempted rape. Not only families and friends of a victim will react to the tragic news but the crisis affects communities. The following attempted rape–murder produced a community reaction.[4]

> It was a shocking, senseless murder. A brutal crime that left Cambridge suspicious and afraid . . . . It was about 5:40 P.M. and [she] was walking home from Radcliffe. . . . As she approached Longfellow Park, along historic Brattle St., a man walked up to her and began pushing and pulling her into the park. Inside the park, her assailant partially disrobed [her] in what police believed was an attempted rape. And then he took a handgun and shot her in the head . . . . Violent crime has made culture-filled Cambridge a jittery city.

The Confidence Attack

The confidence attack is a more subtle setup than the blitz style just described. In the confidence attack the offender gains access to the victim under false pretenses by using deceit, betrayal, and violence. There is interaction between the assailant and the victim prior to the attack. The offender may know the victim from some other time and place and thus may already have developed some kind of relationship with the victim. Or he may establish a relationship as a prelude to the attack. Often there is quite a bit of conversation between victim and assailant. Like the confidence man, he encourages the victim to trust him and then he betrays this trust. This betrayal may be within a short period of time or it may be over a long period. Three subtypes of the confidence attack will be described.

Capturing the victim by verbal means. In this style there is an effort to strike up a conversation with the victim and to use verbal means of capture rather than physical force. The assailant is unknown to the victim prior to that contact and he tries to

---

[4] Joe Heaney, "He Would Put Killer in Chair," *Boston Herald,* June 1, 1974.

establish a kind of dialogue with the victim ostensibly for a reason acceptable to the victim. Once he gains the person's confidence, however, he betrays that confidence.

Rape. The following case was referred to the Boston Victim Counseling Program, and the newspaper account of the trial provides such a diagnosis of this style of attack.[5]

> The victim . . . told the Judge and a jury of 14 men that she returned to her apartment about 1:30 P.M. on Nov. 23, after spending Thanksgiving Day with friends and relatives . . . . About a half hour later . . . her doorbell rang and she pressed the buzzer, which opened an outer door to the apartment house, because she was expecting a female friend who lived a block away. When she opened her apartment door she was confronted by three men. "One of them had a piece of paper in his hand. He said, 'We have something for you.' I replied, 'No thanks' and tried to shut the door. I saw that one of them had a gun. Another pushed me back into the apartment and threw me on the floor." . . .

Murder and robbery. On occasion the victim's employment situation makes him more vulnerable to violence. This was the case with one taxi driver. The newspaper account of the trial aids in diagnosing the style of attack by verbal means.[6]

> A witness placed a man in the front seat of the cab with the cab driver. The same witness said, "A woman was in the rear seat of the cab." . . . There was testimony that the killer fired one shot, and then then two more: "to make sure he was dead."

Knowing the victim. There are two types of knowing the victim. First are the attacks where the assailant is known to the victim; that is, both parties know each other. The assailant is a neighbor, an acquaintance, a friend, a date, or a relative. The offender uses his relationship with the victim to justify being in the situation. He then deceives the person by not honoring the bounds of the relationship.

There are situations in which only one party knows the other. That is, the assailant knows the victim either through some type of relationship to the family or by reading about the person

[5] Alan H. Sheehan, "Rape Victim Identifies in Court Three Roxbury Men as Assailants," *Boston Evening Globe,* June 5, 1974.

[6] Joe Heaney, "She Knows First-Hand about Killing," *Boston Herald,* June 5, 1974.

such as in the newspaper. Two cases illustrate each type of knowing the victim.

Murder and robbery. The relationship was the prime factor in allowing the assailant to gain access to the victim in the following case. Both parties knew each other. The assailant had been fired from his employment with the victim 6 months prior to the murder. The newspaper account was as follows.[7]

> Police believe robbery was the motive in the violent death of a prominent semiretired physician, whose battered body was found by local police in his home . . . . there was evidence of a violent struggle in the room. A piece of electric cord was found around the victim's neck.

Attempted kidnapping and attempted murder. The second type in the category of knowing the victim is where only one party knows the other; obviously it is the assailant. The case described here was initially planned as a kidnapping but the assailant was confronted with the unexpected presence of another person. Therefore, there were two victims to this case.

> It was 9 P.M. on a September evening. The son of a well-known and prominent wealthy family was waiting for his brother to come to his house. The doorbell rang and the man opened the door expecting his brother. Instead, a man wearing a baseball cap pulled down to his ears extended a gun and said, "Open the door and let me in."
>
> Once inside, the assailant realized there was another person present and asked, "Who is he?" The man replied that it was his father-in-law. The assailant had not anticipated this and warned that if anyone else were in the house and they lied about it, he would kill everyone.
>
> The assailant handcuffed and blindfolded the young man and then put the gun down to tie up the older man. In this time period, the younger man fell upon the gun and managed to pick it up between his hands and fired it at the assailant. The shot hit the assailant, who then lunged for the young man who managed to throw himself at the assailant with success. With this, the assailant left the house, leaving behind the briefcase with the details of the ransom note.

Kidnapping cases have different components from rape and murder cases in that very often the planned details of the crime may be determined. In this case, the ransom note revealed the full

[7] *The Aegis*, Bel Air, Md., August 17, 1967.

intent of the kidnapper. For example, it was learned that the assailant had spent 3 months researching kidnapping cases in the Library of Congress. This attempt was his second try. In this situation, it was learned that one of the assailant's sisters had attended school with the victim's sister. The kidnapper had seen a newspaper picture of the victim's mother following her husband's casket and a story stating that the victim's father had died and left substantial sums of money to his children. The ransom note identified the victim's mother as the person who would be contacted. Elaborate directions as to the manner in which the phone call would be enacted were given with the final direction, "If you do not cooperate, there will be a picture of you following your son's casket."

As the victim scene developed, it became apparent that the assailant intended to murder the father-in-law whom the assailant had not expected to be there. It was only the young man's ability to act defensively in the situation that saved both lives. It was speculated from the ransom note that the victim was to be buried alive and would have died if the kidnapping instructions were not followed.

Controlling the victim over time. There are situations where the offender uses the crime as a means to control people, not for just the one incident but over a long period of time. In rape, the woman may be an ex-girl friend or an ex-wife of the offender and he assumes he still has full sexual rights with her. These victims are beaten and threatened with their life, as well as sexually assaulted.

Rape and assault. This situation involved a mother, her son, and her girlfriend. She said,

> It was in the middle of the night and he snuck in through the window—he has done it before and there have been violent scenes. He thinks he can get away with this even though we have been separated 5 years and the divorce is pending. He knows it upsets the kids but he keeps doing it. Well, I was screaming and yelling and he wouldn't stop. At one point I ran into the living room and he followed and then he saw Joan, my girlfriend who was staying overnight. He said, "Oh, you are going to join in too." She was so scared but he threatened to hurt the kids so she came into the room . . . .

This case was reported to the police and the charges of rape could be filed against the assailant by the girlfriend of the wife but the wife was only allowed to file assault charges. The 3-year-old son developed symptoms of insomnia, nightmares, and kept crying "Go away," which is what the mother yelled to the father. The child developed a 104° F temperature and the decision was made to place him in a foster home until the family situation was remedied.

Murder. There are situations in which betrayal of either the relationship or the activities involved in the relationship can culminate in a violent crime. Extortion and blackmail perhaps may be viewed as lesser violent means of dealing with the betrayal. The following case, however, which is described in more detail later in this chapter, involved the murder of the boyfriend of the client who was in a counseling situation with the nurse–therapist. The client said:

> Mark was selling drugs and importing drugs from Canada. He lived with some druggies who also were involved. Mark was arrested by the federal agents and told if he would be a witness to his housemates, who had long records of drug charges, he would receive a lighter sentence. He agreed to this but his housemate found out and shot him.

FAMILY REACTION TO HOMICIDE[8]

The Acute Grief Phase

Families of homicide victims experience a two-phase trauma reaction: the acute crisis and the reorganization phase. The crisis phase consists of an acute grief process including immediate reactions to the homicide, the funeral details, thoughts about the assailant, and the police investigation. In listening to families talk of their immediate reactions to the tragedy, two thoughts are noted: their loss of the family member (ego-oriented thought) and their horror for the manner in which the family member died (victim-oriented thought). Following this immediate reaction, families begin to ask a series of questions.

Ego-oriented thoughts. For many, the news of the homicide is a severe blow to the ego. Losing a significant person leaves uppermost in their mind their own personal loss. One brother said, "I never felt so overwhelmed with emptiness before; it was

[8]The following sections are reprinted with permission from A. W. Burgess, "Family Reaction to Homicide," *Amer. J. Orthopsychiatry*, **45**, No. 3 (1975), 391–398. Copyright 1975, the American Journal of Orthopsychiatry.

as though someone cut my insides out." The somatic analogy reflects the tremendous impact implying that a part of the self has been lost through the victim's death. Or the survivor may react to the untimely and unexpected nature of the news. One widower talked of his reaction to people in general:

> It is hard enough to accept natural death, but it's worse with violent death. It's so abrupt. So shocking. It's hard to trust people.

Victim-oriented thoughts. Homicide is the killing of one human being by another. People are especially concerned about the physical injury inflicted on the victim specific to the brutality of the assailant and the varying degrees of trauma associated with the death. The assailant's method of killing may become a preoccupation, and include concern about the victim's suffering. One person said:

> I mentally tried to put myself in my brother's position. Did he fight? How much agony did he go through?

Who Did It?

There is an urgency to wanting to know the facts: who did it; who is the murderer? These questions correlate with the style of attack, the way in which the assailant gained access to the victim. The style may then determine if the victim knew the assailant, if it was a confidence attack or if it was a blitz attack.

Blitz murder: the stranger. If there is no suspect, the family must give considerable energy in working with the police to help determine leads and to reconstruct the victim's life prior to the homicide, and to help reconstruct events during and following the murder.

The blitz style of attack is very difficult to come to terms with when trying to find some reason for the murder. As cited in the first case, the widow spoke of the murder as being a case of "mistaken identity."

Confidence murder; assailant initiates interaction. The interaction or relationship that a homicide victim has with the assailant adds a complicated dimension to the dynamics of the case. One daughter said, "I can accept my father's death but not the way in which he died." This style of attack was captured over time.

The father was murdered by contract and his family, except
for the daughter, had resigned themselves to his violent death by
the Mafia.

When an assailant with an established relationship is also
known to the family, the family has to deal with their feelings
about their own relationship with the assailant.

In cases where the style of attack is not clear-cut and the assailant is never apprehended, there is no feeling of closure to the
crime. Families have been known to go through the incident themselves as part of the settlement process. For example, one family
went as a unit to the deserted area in the country where the
daughter's body was found and tried to act out the scene. A cousin said,

> I tried to imagine how he did it and why she couldn't get away . . .
> she must have been in so much pain . . . I can't stand to think about
> it . . . . This might sound morbid to you but it was just something
> I had to do.

What Can I Do?

One of the immediate reactions families describe is a wish to
do something physically about the crime. An overwhelming feeling
of helplessness may trigger this wish for action, usually against the
assailant; however, strict limits are placed on people taking matters
into their own hands. National attention has been given to one rape
victim who sought out her assailant and shot him. The result of her
actions was her conviction for second-degree murder.[9]

Families will often describe feelings of outrage, anger, and aggression toward the assailant. The father of a murdered daughter
said, "I am overwhelmed with rage. I would kill him if I could." A
brother who talked of his tremendous feelings of revenge repeated
how he wished to "get his hands on the guy." Later during the
trial the brother became preoccupied with the defendant's hands
and said:

> I sat there and looked at his hands, . . . remembering what he did. I
> wished so much that he would come near me. I wanted to choke him
> to death and I really wanted him to come near me so I would have
> the chance.

[9] L. Fosburgh, "Woman Convicted in ' Rape Slaying,' *Los Angeles Sunday
Herald Advertiser*, October 6, 1974.

What Do I Do Now?

The next set of questions that arises regard those reality issues the family must complete. Homicide includes all the activities that are part of the grieving process, including funeral or memorial services.

Notification of others. In a natural death, the family and friends take responsibility for notifying other people of the death and the funeral plans. A homicide, however, usually receives media coverage that may further complicate the grieving process. One family complained of receiving "weird letters and crank calls' because of all the publicity given the murder. One niece reported the following:

> The news was on television immediately . . . . I couldn't stand all the phone calls and people saying such dumb things as, "that couldn't be your uncle that was murdered, was it. What happened?" Who did they think it was with his name, occupation, and address blared out with all the details?

Viewing the victim. Someone has to identify the body; this can place an added psychological burden on a family member to whom the task falls. In one family, it was the daughter who was the only person who felt psychologically strong enough. She said when the police first told her the news, she screamed. When she had to identify her father she was sick to her stomach.

Funeral activities. One of the duties that occupies the family's time in the first week following a homicide is attending to the funeral details and arrangements. Such decisions as whether to have an open casket must be made. This may depend on the physical appearance of the body and can be a difficult decision for the family. Families must take into account how newspaper reporting has handled the situation in terms of what peoples' fantasies might be. Families must also consider the wishes, if they are known, of the victim. In one case, the victim had previously requested having an open casket when he died. This wish heavily influenced the family decision even though the victim had been badly beaten and bruised.

So much activity surrounds the first week after receiving the news that people may not show an emotional reaction until after the funeral. A daughter reported this as follows:

I had to go to the state where it happened. It was exhausting. When I went to the police, they talked and talked and talked and I had to tell all I know. I had to see pictures of the scene. He was slumped over in the car. I had to identify the car and then go to the morgue and identify the body. Had to claim the body and sign papers. Had to make all the funeral arrangements. Had to buy a suit, shoes and such for my father. Had to write the notice for the newspaper. Then there were more questions by the police and FBI. Then I had to buy clothes for my family and go to the airport and pick them up . . . . The funeral was a long drive and in the car it really hit me . . . . My grandmother started it by saying, "God, don't burn my baby." That really hit me . . . me . . . . I don't remember anything after that . . . Except in the chapel I remember the body going into the furnace or knowing it was going in there. It was my father's wish . . . . My grandmother started up again.

Physical signs and symptoms. Families are numb and confused and will describe a number of physical concerns. Insomnia, sleep pattern disturbances, headaches, chest pain, palpitations, and gastrointestinal upsets are quite common. Very often sedatives and tranquilizers are prescribed in an attempt to relieve the physical symptoms. People will describe not feeling or remembering much about the first weeks and even months.

REACTIONS OVER TIME: REORGANIZATION PHASE

Two major themes were noted in the reorganization period following the acute grief period. Families have to deal with their own psychological reactions and they have to deal with the sociolegal issues involved with the crime of homicide.

Psychological Issues

Grief work. The family has to go through the process of grief work. This is the psychological process that moves the person from being preoccupied with thoughts of the lost person, through painful recollections of the loss experience, to the final step of settling the loss as an integrative experience.[10] In describing the feeling of loss, one person said:

[10] C. Parkes, *Bereavement: Studies of Grief in Adult Life* (New York: International Universities Press, (1972), p. 77.

It is an awful loss that doesn't strike home for weeks and then the feeling of loss and wondering how to pick up the pieces.

Reviewing memories of the victim, as part of grief work, is noted with one widower:

It was all sort of life from the movie, Love Story, the way things turned out. And now the only.thing I can do is forget. . . . I can't go on thinking about it.

Contrasting the victim with the crime is a theme noted in various families. Many people talk of the contrast between the violent act committed to the victim and the victim's nonaggressive nature. One widow said, "He hated violence . . . and he died by it."

Settlement of the "if only" reaction is important to some people. As the families learn the details of the homicide, they begin to say "If only I had done such and such, this would not have happened." One person said, "If only I had stayed one more day, this never would have happened." The London Study on bereavement discusses the expression of self-reproachful ideas similar to "if only."[11]

Dreams and nightmares. Dreaming of the lost person in terms of wish fulfillment is documented in bereavement studies.[12] Wish-fulfillment dreams are seen in survivors in terms of trying to save the victim. One person described a dream in which she tried to warn her cousin not to go with the murderer and woke up in the middle of the dream crying. Another person described the following dream in which he tried unsuccessfully to save his brother.

They were vivid dreams where I would be struggling. I was fighting and bouncing all over and would see the murder room and I would see my brother's face and it would be all contorted. I'd be in it and I couldn't move—I wasn't able to do anything. Then I would wake up and not be able to go back to sleep . . . that was eating me up . . . had them especially after a bad day.

Phobic reactions. As with rape victims, phobic reactions are common with family members and develop according to the specific circumstances surrounding the events of the crime. One sister

[11] Ibid.
[12] Ibid.

of an unsolved murder victim developed the fear of having people walk behind her, including her own boyfriend.

Families become very aware of the potential for a crime occurring and cope by adding protective measures. Many families will take special precautions to protect themselves. Men will obtain permits to carry guns or will have guns at their bedside. Many people will put burglar alarms in their homes.

Identification with tragedy. Identification with the dead person was noted as one way people dealt with the painful loss. One sister immediately began sleeping in her dead sister's bed and wearing her clothes. Widows, specifically, would identify with other women whose husbands had been murdered. These women talked of having something in common with Jacqueline Onassis, Ethel Kennedy, and Coretta King. Or, in the case of a patrolman's wife, the remark was made, "She has joined the 'group'."

Role change. Death forces people into sudden role changes for which they have little preparation. Loss of a wife changes a husband to a widower; loss of an only child or an only uncle or only cousin can totally eliminate the role the survivor held. Being forced into assuming a new identity and giving up an important role adds a difficult dimension to the grief process.

Socio-Legal Issues

The court process. All homicide cases will involve some degree of police and court procedure. There will be investigations to find the murderer. This entire process has a major effect on the grief reaction and crisis settlement. There are many feelings evoked during the process but one of the hardest to bear, if the case goes to court, is the impersonal attitude of court and the participants. One person described it clearly:

> . . . Here was a doctor . . . his life snuffed out and it was treated so casually . . . . Like, so what . . . . People forget . . . so much time elapses.

Concept of blame. Murder undermines one's faith in the world as an ordered and secure place. Studies show that untimely natural deaths shake confidence in this sense of security. Blaming someone for a tragedy is a less disturbing alternative than facing the fact that life is uncertain. It allows people to continue to be in control by putting the responsibility onto another person. Not to be able to explain a situation makes people feel helpless.

People look for a target to project their feelings. The main target is usually the assailant. Families want justice and the assailant prosecuted. Some people believe in capital punishment; others see prison as the punishment for his unlawful actions. Some people state that the assailant is a "sick" person and should be psychiatrically treated because they "don't want him to harm anyone else."

Another target is the criminal justice system. Families can become angry at the police for being unsuccessful in finding the assailant. Other people focus on the court process and become angry at the judges for "letting criminals right out the door after they are apprehended." Society is also a target for blame. One widower said:

> I am a conservative by nature but this has made me somewhat of a radical. . . . to think the society you live in produced a guy like that.

And not infrequently the victim may be blamed. This concept is described in the literature as *victim-precipitation* and *victim-participation*.[13] This concept holds that no victim is entirely innocent but rather participates to some degree in the crime.

SPECIAL INTERVENTION SITUATIONS

There is a conscious need by people to settle the incident, to make some sense out of what happened, to explain it to themselves, to classify it along with other life events, and to make it somehow "fit" into their reorganized life-style. Families who had adequate emotional support through a social network or through crisis counseling tend to have a good chance of settling the acute crisis period and dealing with the long-term reactions. There are some people, however, who will have difficulty in settling the trauma syndrome because of the manner in which outside people treat them in regard to the situation. One case is where people *deliberately* avoid the family, and consequently, are not supportive. The second situation is where people *unwittingly* avoid the family and thus no support is offered.

[13] M. Amir, "Victim Precipitated Forcible Rape," *Journal of Criminal Law* 58 (1967), 493.

Deliberate Avoidance by Social Matrix

To be acknowledged as a victim involves people validating the crime as a crime. One category in which people have considerable ambivalence over viewing a crime as a bonafide crime often occurs in the style of attack: controlled over time. In such situations, the victim has a long-standing relationship of some type with the murderer or assailant.

In the following case, the victim belonged to a drug ring and because he "squealed" to the federal agents, he received little recognition as a human being who had died. Subsequently the girl friend had great difficulty grieving because no one acknowledged that her boy friend was "worth it." The girl friend of the victim was treated by a nurse–therapist who had been seeing the couple prior to the murder and the total case is described as follows.

Lori, a 16-year-old adolescent woman, and her 27-year-old boyfriend Mark came to the community health center for pregnancy counseling. Together they had decided that the best alternative for them would be for Lori to have an abortion. Since Lori was a minor, she needed parental permission for a legal abortion. Her parents were divorced and she lived with her mother. The mother did not want to be involved in family counseling but stated she would be willing to give her permission for the abortion. Mark became Lori's sole support system. He was very helpful emotionally and financially through the abortion process.

Lori and Mark returned for three sessions of post-abortion counseling. At this time, Mark requested to see the nurse individually to "talk over some things."

The nurse saw him twice before he was murdered. He was very much involved in "dealing"—selling drugs, especially speed—and he also described main-lining speed. He talked of feeling confused and ambivalent about his life-style and especially wanted to talk about what he might change in himself. When he did not keep his last appointment, the nurse called him at home. He responded, "There are some heavy things going on here; I'll call you back." He never did call. He was shot in the heart by one of his housemates that afternoon.

Lori contacted the nurse after the murder and expressed her request to talk things over. The nurse saw Lori for crisis counseling for several sessions. The following are her reactions to a sequence of events.

Initial reaction: "I can't believe I lost him." Lori was especially angry toward the housemates and said, "Those druggies make me furious." This reaction was in contrast to her prior feeling in that she rather enjoyed the life-style they led. Lori now said she did not want to have anything to do with them.

Lori said there was no one for her to talk to; her mother was just not interested. Her peers were very inquisitive but not supportive. They just wanted to talk of the murder and not of how she was feeling about her loss.

One of her fears was that the housemates might come after her. She said she was really afraid to talk to anyone but found she had to talk to someone. She had received a phone call warning her not to talk to the police.

Case analysis of crisis intervention. Lori had a strong need to know the entire story and why Mark was killed even if that meant going to the narcotic agent. She talked this over with the therapist, decided to go, and was very glad she did. She was relieved to be able to trust someone with her information. She learned the facts of the case. Mark was importing drugs from Canada and selling them. He was arrested by federal agents and told if he would testify against his housemates who had long histories of drug charges, he would receive a lighter sentence. Mark agreed to do this. However, his housemate found out and shot him in the heart.

Lori agreed to testify at the probable cause hearing in court even though she was very frightened. This bothered her because she said, "I felt more frightened for myself than upset for Mark." Other people looked on her as a "rat" and she found this difficult to deal with.

When all the people involved were in jail, Lori returned to the house where the murder had occurred. She said, "I could see the whole thing happen as I stood there . . . it was dreadful but real for me."

Lori struggled with two "if only" thoughts: If only Mark had come to see her that fatal afternoon and if only Mark had kept his appointment with the therapist.

There were several changes in life-style following the murder. Lori moved from her apartment to her mother's house for several months. She isolated herself from people and said, "I can't stand to answer all their busybody questions and they really don't care. They just want the goods." There was no memorial service for Mark but Lori went regularly to the grave. She said, "I bring flowers; I talk to Mark and I cry." She expressed her grief at graveside and with the therapist.

This case illustrates the therapeutic influence that crisis intervention has when the murder victim is not socially acknowledged. The girlfriend had no one in her social network to help her grieve and settle the crisis experience. She did seek out the therapist who had helped her with a previous crisis, the abortion. Crisis counseling was initiated and she was able to reorganize her lifestyle after several months. Her words indicating an adequate level of settlement, verified with the strengths noted in her behavior, were "I've woken up to the world and I am better for it."

Unwitting Avoidance by Social Matrix

There are situations in which a murder or other crime may well be acknowledged, but for some reason the family receives no support in dealing with the crisis. The following case illustrates the need for clinicians who do crisis intervention to initiate services rather than waiting for clients to seek them out. This case, shows how a family was immobilized and unable to seek any type of crisis services.[14]

> Pam, a 21-year-old student, was presented at an outpatient psychiatric community clinic following referral from the Student Health service. As she talked during the interview, she would periodically dig her fingernails into her palms and she acknowledged having cut her arm on several occasions.

> Pam talked of having had feelings of "falling apart" and of not being able to control herself but that she currently felt more in control of her behavior. She felt that her difficulties were caused by her being away from home for the first time. She would become upset, however, when she went home because "mother is so sad and father so old."

> Pam almost immediately began talking about her sister's death and murder 6 years previously. She did this with a great deal of intense emotion, explaining that it was very difficult for her to talk about it because they had been very close, with the sister being a "mother" to her.

> Historically, mother did not notice Pam's childhood problems, but her sister did and tried to help her. Pam views herself as having been a tomboy (because father had wanted a boy and Pam had tried to please him), fat, very self-conscious, shy, and ugly because of a severe acne problem. The sister began helping Pam by getting her to lose weight and was about to take her to a dermatologist when she was murdered.

> The nurse asked Pam to describe the events relevant to the murder. The sister went to work as usual the morning after a holiday. The

---

[14.]This case is adapted from A. W. Burgess and A. Lazare, *Psychiatric Nursing in the Hospital and the Community,* Second Edition (Englewood Cliffs, N. J.: Prentice-Hall, Inc., 1976.)

employer called the home around 10 A.M. to find out where she was. The family became concerned and called the police, who felt it was not that serious a concern for alarm at 11 A.M. but stated they would begin a search. The father went to retrace the daughter's usual path to work. The father found his daughter strangled with her stocking in an isolated field that was part of the shortcut she often took to go to work.

Pam wept at this point and said that the feelings she had were of hatred and these feelings were difficult for her to think about as they upset her so much. The resentful feelings she had were toward the police department, who wouldn't respond quickly to look for her sister; then when the father did find the body, they sent their rookies to "mess up the clues so that the murderer was never found."

The hatred feelings were also for the townspeople who made the family feel like "freaks" and forced them to withdraw, as a family, into their house "like strange animals in a cage." The family did receive a lot of crank calls and weird letters at the time and people continually talked about the incident in the town.

Pam saw this as the reason for her subsequent withdrawal from social contacts (she had one girlfriend) and for not dating in high school. Pam could recall feeling "numb" at the funeral and remembered looking at people to see their reaction. She then recalled her grandfather's funeral when she was seven when she did the same thing and they had to take her out of the church. She did not cry at the time of her sister's death but about 2 years later when a person whom she liked very much died, she cried with great feeling, realizing then that she was also weeping for her sister.

After the sister's death, Pam slept in her sister's bed (Pam's had been the lower part of a trundle bed) and she wore her sister's clothes. Her sister had been 2 years older than Pam.

Pam frequently had nightmares about a man coming in the window with a knife to stab her and had to receive medication from a local physician before these stopped. These nightmares developed into a fear that she had continued to have where she would not allow anyone to walk behind her, including her boyfriend. She had been to her sister's grave only twice in the 6-year period.

Case analysis of unresolved homicide grief.   One can readily make the diagnosis that the patient is suffering from an unresolved homicide grief for two reasons:

1. The patient is unable to discuss with equanimity a death that occurred 6 years previously. With a supportive listener, she immediately began to discuss the death with intense emotion.
2. There was a history of failure to grieve at the time of the death.

As to the reasons for her inability to grieve, the client suggests that it was because she and her sister had been very close, with the sister being a "mother" to her. This closeness is further illustrated by the patient sleeping in the sister's bed and wearing her clothes. In addition, the patient has nightmares that she too is being murdered. It becomes clear that the failure to grieve is related to some quality regarding the relationship between the patient and her sister. The data suggests two hypotheses. First, although the client verbalizes positive feelings toward the sister, she must have harbored many negative feelings toward someone who received from the mother what the patient did not. In effect, besides loving the sister, the client hated her. The death consequently evoked too much guilt to let the client grieve. Digging her fingernails into her palms and cutting her arm on several occasions was a means of relieving guilt. As an alternative hypothesis, it may be postulated that the client was so attached to the sister, as the only one who cared, that to grieve would be to acknowledge that the sister really died. By not grieving, the sister is somehow still alive.

Whichever hypothesis is correct, the therapist must provide a supportive relationship that will allow the client to mourn her sister. In the process, the therapist will discover and help the client realize and understand the nature of the relationship to the sister that made the grief process so difficult.

SUMMARY

The increase in violence in our society will undoubtedly place added demands on mental health facilities, who are called upon to provide services to victims and their families. This chapter describes crimes of murder, rape, and attempted kidnapping and murder within a typology for the style of attack. Two styles of attack are identified as *blitz* and *confidence*, with three subtypes under the confidence attack.

Family reactions to homicide of a family member reveal a two-phased syndrome. The crisis phase consists of an acute grief process including immediate reactions to the homicide, the questions about the assailant, the funeral details, and the police investigation. The long-term reorganization phase include the psychological issues of bereavement and the socio-legal issues of the criminal justice system.

Two specific intervention situations are discussed in terms of case illustrations of helping the person grieve when the victim has been socially excluded and a case where unresolved homicide grief occurred as a result of no crisis intervention and lack of social network support.

12

aggressive sexual offenders: diagnosis and treatment

by A. Nicholas Groth, Ph.D., and Murray L. Cohen, Ph.D.

Chapter 11 dealt with physical violence and the family reactions to the homicide of one of its members. Physical sexual violence is another alarming social problem which appears to be on the increase. Chapter 12 deals with the issue of sexual assault—specifically rape—from the standpoint of the offender, and Chapter 13 will consider the topic in regard to the victim. This chapter presents some of the observations and results of 15 years of clinical work in studying the dangerous male sexual offender.

RAPE: THE OFFENSE

Rape is legally defined as sexual intercourse or unnatural sexual intercourse by a person with another person who is compelled to submit by force and against his or her will or by threat of bodily injury.[1] Rape, then, is *any* form of sexual assault. It is

Dr. Groth is Chief Psychologist, Massachusetts Department of Mental Health, Division of Legal Medicine.

Dr. Cohen is Professor of Psychology and Chairman of the Clinical-Community Psychology program at Boston University.

[1]Massachusetts Session Laws, Chapter 474, Section 7, July 3, 1974.

forcing a person to submit to and/or to commit a sexual act against his or her will through intimidation, threat, and/or physical force. It is a *sexual offense* punishable by imprisonment "for life or for any term of years."[2] It is an offense usually committed by men against women, children, and other men.

It is also a *sexual deviation*. Although not listed in the *Diagnostic Manual* of the American Psychiatric Association and generally ignored in texts of abnormal psychology, rape is in fact a sexual deviation in the truest sense of the word: it is sexual behavior in the service of nonsexual needs. Contrary to popular belief forcible rape is *not* motivated *primarily* by a need for sexual gratification, and the misconception that it is has led to the curious state of affairs in which the victim is often regarded as more responsible for the crime than the offender, and the existence of emotional problems in the offender that require psychological remedy go unnoticed and neglected.

Until recently very little has been known about the psychology of rape, and even today our knowledge is incomplete. One reason for this is that rather than seeking professional help, the rapist *acts out* his emotional problems; that is, he attempts to relieve the psychological stresses and pressures he is experiencing through the act of rape. *Acting-out* is "manifesting the purposive behavior appropriate to an older situation in a new situation which symbolically represents it."[3] In other words, unresolved conflicts in the psychological development of the offender lie behind and give rise to the symptom of rape. Self-referral to a mental health agency is uncharacteristic of the rapist since he feels compelled to discharge the emotional turmoil he is caught up in behaviorally. It is through the desperate act of rape that he tries to free himself of his psychological distress. In addition, the offender feels that to face what is going on within him will result in his destruction. Again and again the answer to "Why didn't you seek some help with your problems before you acted out?" has been "I was afraid I'd wind up in prison or in the 'bug house'." Not only then does the rapist not come to the attention of mental health practitioners through self-referral but also once he acts out and is apprehended, he is processed through the criminal justice system and is sent to a correctional institution. There usually are inadequate psychological services in such institutions and the climate within a prison works against motivating the rapist to take advantage of any available mental health program. To reveal that you

[2] Ibid., Section 22.

[3] H. English and A. English *A Comprehensive Dictionary of Psychological and Psychoanalytical Terms* (New York: Longmans, Green and Co., 1958).

are a sexual offender may put your life in danger from other inmates. Even when this is not so, the correctional system itself, which places a premium on conformity and passivity, is not conducive to psychological rehabilitation. For these reasons then, little has been known about rape and much confusion continues to surround this form of sexual psychopathy. A serious irony has evolved: By going to prison the rapist's psychological problems are not treated and he continues to constitute a risk to the community when he is released; at the same time, by going to prison he does not come to the attention of mental health professionals and, therefore, they do not have the opportunity to develop an expertise in regard to the diagnosis and treatment of such individuals. Lacking such skills, mental health practitioners are then reluctant to accept professional responsibility for the rapist and are content to allow him to be dealt with by agencies other than those of the Department of Mental Health. In regarding the rapist as a felon rather than as a patient, punishment rather than treatment occurs. The result is that the rapist returns to the community (unless he serves a life sentence or dies in prison) ill-equipped to manage the emotional demands of his life differently than he did when he committed his offense. Imprisonment has done nothing to lesson the danger he constitutes to society. It will not deter him from repeating the offense and it will only prevent him from coming to the attention of those professionals who specialize in the detection and amelioration of psychological disturbance.

This societal self-perpetuating and self-defeating state of events was, in part at least, interrupted in Massachusetts in 1958 with the enactment of special legislation which created a Center for the Diagnosis and Treatment of Sexually Dangerous Persons.[4] A "sexually dangerous person" was defined as "any person whose misconduct in sexual matters indicates a general lack of power to control his sexual impulses, as evidenced by repetitive or compulsive behavior and either violence, or aggression by an adult against a victim under the age of 16 years, and who, as a result, is likely to attack or otherwise inflict injury on the objects of his uncontrolled or uncontrollable desires."[5]

The statute provides for the diagnostic study, at the discretion of the Court, of any person *convicted* of any of a number of

[4]Massachusetts General Laws, Chapter 646, Acts 1958, Chapter 123A. Amendments: Chapter 615, Acts 1959, Section 2, Chapter 123A; Chapter 347, Acts 1960, Section 9, Chapter 123A; Chapter 608, Acts 1966, Section 9, Chapter 123A.

[5]Massachusetts General Laws, Chapter 123A, Section 1.

specified sexual offenses[6] and (if adjudicated to be "sexually dangerous") for an indefinite civil commitment (from a minimum of 1 day to a maximum of that person's natural life) either in lieu of or in addition to his prison sentence.[7] This statute came into being as the direct result of a shocking sexual murder of two pre-adolescent boys by a man who had been released from prison only a short time before, at the expiration of his sentence for sexually attacking and almost killing another young boy several years earlier. It became tragically clear that imprisonment alone was inadequate and ineffective in protecting the public from such dangerous offenders and so the Massachusetts Treatment Center came into existence. The Center[8] itself is operated under the joint jurisdiction of the Department of Mental Health, which is responsible for the psychiatric care of the patient, and the Department of Correction, which is responsible for the physical care of the patient and the maintenance of security. As described by a Justice of the Federal District Court, the Treatment Center "is by no means simply a place for the segregation and confinement of sexually dangerous persons, but rather one where they receive continuous rehabilitative treatment by a professional staff of psychiatrists, psychologists, and social workers."[9] This law, then, permits the indefinite confinement of a convicted sexual offender for as long as he continues to constitute a physical danger to the community with the provision that while thus incarcerated he be afforded psychological treatment (psychotherapy) to help him resolve those problems that result in his being a danger to others. This law succeeded then in bringing the rapist to the attention of mental health professionals, and a body of information as to the psychological meanings of his offenses and the origins of his behavior have at last begun to be developed. "Sexual dangerous-

[6]These crimes include indecent assault and battery; rape; carnal knowledge and abuse of a child under 16; assault with intent to rape; open and gross lewdness and lascivious behavior; incest; sodomy; buggery; unnatural and lascivious acts with another; lewd, wanton, and lascivious behavior; indecent exposure; or attempts to commit any of the above.

[7]For a detailed explanation of this law see E. Powers, *The Basic Structure of the Administration of Criminal Justice in Massachusetts,* 6th edition (Boston: Massachusetts Correctional Association, 1973), Chapter 8.

[8]For a detailed description of this facility, see H. L. Kozol, M. L. Cohen, and R. F. Garofalo "The Criminally Dangerous Sex Offender," *New England Journal of Medicine,* Vol. 275 (July 1966), and/or A. L. McGarry and R. D. Cotton, "A Study in Civil Commitment: The Massachusetts Sexually Dangerous Persons Act," *Harvard Journal on Legislation,* Vol. 6, 1969.

[9] Meola v. Fitzpatrick, 322 Federal Supplement 878, 1971.

ness," then, is a legal, not a psychiatric, diagnosis. Clinically, it amounts to a prediction of behavior which may occur across the whole spectrum of conventional psychiatric nosology and which may be symptomatic of psychological disorders that are neurotic, characterological, or psychotic in nature. Since this concept of "sexual dangerousness" involves homogeneous symptoms of heterogeneous origins, it is difficult to be very definitive about the identification and treatment of such a condition. We shall attempt, however, to present our state of knowledge to date regarding the psychology of the dangerous sexual offender and to describe the treatment program that has evolved based on our understanding of the dynamics of this pathology.

The subjects of our work consist of more than 300 male adults committed to the Treatment Center since its inception. These are men who have sexually aggressed against adults or children and have inflicted, attempted to inflict, or threatened to inflict serious bodily harm on their victims in the course of the sexual assault. Although there is great variation among these offenders with regard to the specific factors and dynamics underlying their offenses, four distinctive patterns of assault emerge.

PATTERNS OF RAPE

Rape, which is defined here as *any* form of forcible sexual assault, is multidetermined. It is motivated by a combination of factors. Contrary to popular belief, however, genital sexuality is *not* the prime factor. Instead, sex becomes the vehicle by which the offender expresses and gratifies other needs and wishes.

Descriptively, the act of rape involves both sexual and aggressive features. It is clear, however, that different relationships between these two components exist and give rise to different patterns of sexual assault.

In some acts of rape the intent of the act is primarily aggressive. Far more physical force is employed by the offender than would be necessary simply to overpower his victim. In this type of assault the victim is brutally attacked, punched, choked, kicked, and beaten. Sexual excitation or erotic feelings on the part of the offender are minimal or nonexistent, and often he must force his victim to masturbate him or to fellate him in order to obtain an erection. It is not sexual gratification he is seeking; it is the humiliation, degradation, and defilement of his victim; and he uses sex to this end. He has developed the attitude that sex is "dirty," and this becomes his weapon, his means of expressing the anger, rage, and resentment that he has been long harboring towards women. Usually in these cases the victim is a stranger or only slightly known to her assailant, and often she is significantly older than he. His attack can be understood only as a displacement of anger from the actual women in his life who aroused it onto a symbolic substitute. It is through the act of rape that this offender vents his rage and seeks to retaliate and revenge himself for perceived wrongs or rejections suffered in his relationships with significant women in his life. The assault is experienced by the offender as the result of an "uncontrollable impulse" and almost always follows some precipitating conflictual or frustrating event involving his wife, girlfriend, or mother. It is readily apparent that the rape is not meant to gratify an intense sexual desire but rather to serve an aggressive, hostile motive.

In other cases of rape the sexual assault appears to be in the service of power and mastery. It is the means by which the offender attempts to prove to himself that he is strong, competent, and "in charge" and to reassure himself as to his adequacy, potency, and desirability as a "man." This assailant has deeply rooted and pervasive feelings of inadequacy, worthlessness, and vulnerability. He is very insecure in regard to his sense of identity, and frequently he is terrified of emerging homosexual impulses. By capturing and placing his victim in a helpless situation—often forcing her to submit through intimidation, threat with a weapon, or by tying her up—he gratifies a need to feel powerful and in control (his victim must now do whatever he wants). Often he has felt under the control of women (mother, wife, etc.); now he has control over another, a woman, who unconsciously represents everything he dislikes about himself and which he wants to overcome: being feminine, being weak, being helpless. There is actually no wish to hurt the victim, and usually this offender uses only whatever force is necessary to overpower or subdue her—generally she is not physically brutalized. In fact this type of offender often hopes that the victim will enjoy the assault. There is always a fantasy-wish operating in this type of rapist that once he overcomes his victim's initial resistance, she will be "turned on" by him, will welcome his sexual embrace, and will be impressed with his sexual prowess and skill. Such a fantasy, so desperately believed by this offender, clearly reflects an effort to compensate for and to counteract feelings of impotency, worthlessness, and inadequacy. Through the act of rape he seeks to deny his homosexual anxieties, to conquer his fear of women, and to assert his manhood by bringing about (in a counterphobic way) a sexual relationship with a woman. Even when he succeeds in his assault—for many of these offenders fail to complete the rape and are often convicted of "indecent assault" or "assault with intent to rape"—he is not relieved of his doubts and typically feels compelled to repeat his offenses again and again, each series of rapes being precipitated in this offender by some perceived challenge by a female or threat by a male.

In still other cases, both sexual and aggressive needs become components of a single psychological experience: sadism. This offender is not able to experience or even fantasize sexual desires without a concomitant arousal of aggressive thoughts and feelings. Such an offender is frequently impotent with women until there is resistance; then he becomes sexually aroused and the more the woman resists, the more excited he becomes and the more excited he becomes, the more aggressive he becomes. In the act of rape, the sexual excitation appears to depend on the presence of force or aggression and, in turn, aggression itself has an erotic quality associated with it. Aggression may be eroticized to the point that, in extreme cases, the sexual abuse of the victim results in a "lust murder." In most cases the sadistic quality of this offender's sexuality is projected onto the victim and he sees her screams, protestations, and struggle not as a refusal but as an expression of her own sexual excitement and pleasure.

Finally, there are cases in which rape appears to be motivated by a sense of narcissistic entitlement in which neither sexuality nor aggression appears to play a dominant role. Neither of these impulses is present to any degree of intensity and the act can be best understood in the context of a general psychopathy as impulsive, stimulus-bound, reactive behavior characteristic of an antisocial personality disorder. The victim is not experienced by the offender in any interpersonal manner. Rather the act appears as simply another aspect of the offender's predatory nature. The rape is frequently carried out in the context of some other antisocial act such as robbery or theft. In such instances the victim is unfortunately present and is exploited sexually. The act is opportunistic, narcissistic, and impulsive. It is another form of stealing, of taking something on impulse by a person who is characteristically exploitative in his relationship to the world and who places a premium on sexuality and aggression in regard to self-definition.

In *every* case of rape there are components of *all* the features described above. In any given instance of rape, displaced, compensatory, sadistic, and narcissistic qualities are discernible, but usually one of these factors is more prominent than others. In addition, there are also unique dynamics involved in specific forms of rape, such as child assault, gang assault, and homosexual rape.

SPECIFIC TYPES OF RAPE

Child Rape

Descriptively, child rape is the forcible sexual assault of an under-aged victim. The selection of a child appears to be multideter-mined. The offender may feel more adequate in dealing with a child than with an adult. It is easier to exploit the child since the child does not pose as much of a physical or psychological threat as does an adult. The offender himself may be an extremely immature and inadequate person who identifies more with a child than with an adult. In some cases, the child may symbolically represent everything the offender negatively feels about himself, and the rape may in part serve to punish the victim for the offender's self-hatred and guilt. Fortunately, the aggressive child rapist is not as common as the more passive child offender whose sexual contact with the child involves pregenital sexual play without aggression. This latter type of pedophile is a nuisance, but generally—especially when the encounter is not ongoing but rather an isolated occurrence and when the offender is a stranger—he is not a serious threat to the physical or psychological[10] safety of the child.

Some child offenders have fixated exclusively on children as their victim-choice since their own adolescence; whereas in other offenders the selection of a child appears to be a regression from a higher level of sexual adaptation. This regression may occur in regard to the age of the victim (from an adult to an adolescent, or to a prepubertal child) and/or the sex of the victim (from an adult heterosexual relationship to the assault of a male adolescent, for example). It is an interesting finding, however, that in our many years of clinical work we have not encountered a regression from an adult homosexual orientation. Those offenders who select underaged males either have done so exclusively since puberty, having no interest or experience with adult

[10] J. Gagnon and W. Simon, "The Child Molester: Surprising Advice for Worried Parents," *Redbook* (February 1969).

sexual relationships of any kind whatsoever, or have done so after having achieved an adult but conflictual heterosexual orientation.

Gang Rape

Descriptively, gang rape refers to the sexual assault of a victim by two or more offenders. A number of factors appear to contribute to the dynamics of this offense. There often appears to be a subtle, unconscious, homosexual factor operating in that a group of males wish to have sex together and use the victim as the vehicle for achieving this. Each man in turn experiences an intense need to prove his manhood to the other group members with considerable anxiety about how the others will regard him. He consequently puts a premium on sexuality and aggression, hurting his victim and forcing degrading sexual acts on her as a way of impressing the other men. A cycle begins in which each offender becomes increasingly brutal and sadistic. Although this varies from situation to situation, it appears that the greater the number of offenders, the greater the degree of violence and aggression on the part of each rapist. Fortunately, more often than not—especially where it involves more than two offenders—this type of rape is not repetitive. That is, it appears that gang rape occurs as the result of a number of psychological and sociocultural factors that are complexly interrelated, and the likelihood of all these factors again reoccurring in exactly the same way is very low. It is not usually the case that these offenders go about committing other rapes as a group.

Homosexual Rape

Descriptively, homosexual rape refers to the forcible sexual assault of one adult male by another. From our experience this appears to be a rare phenomena. In over 3,000 screenings of convicted sexual offenders we have found less than 5 such cases. In all these instances the victim was unknown to the offender. He was usually picked-up while hitchhiking and forced to submit to and/or to perform a sexual act under the threat of a weapon. Sadomasochistic practices usually took place, and the offender in every case suffered from a borderline personality disturbance; his sexual orientation was for the most part homosexual; and the dynamics of sadism seemed most prominent.

The majority of reported cases of homosexual rape have occurred in a prison setting. A study of these offenders by Alan

J. Davis[11] reveals characteristics similar to those reported by us in regard to the heterosexual rapist: The need for sexual release was not the primary motive of the offenders; instead the aim of the assault appeared to be the conquest and degradation of the victim. "Most of the aggressors seem to be members of a subculture that has found most nonsexual avenues of asserting their masculinity closed to them. To them job success, raising a family, and achieving the respect of other men socially have been largely beyond reach. Only sexual and physical prowess stands between them and a feeling of emasculation."[12] When imprisoned, this tenuous sense of identity is undermined and the offender turns to sexual assault to reassure himself of his adequacy and potency. He does not regard himself as a homosexual. The fact that the victim is a male has less to do with the sexual preference of the offender and more to do with environmental circumstances.

MYTHS ABOUT RAPE

The rapist is frequently regarded either as a normal, healthy, "red-blooded" American male who is the victim of a provocative and seductive but punitive woman or as some oversexed, demented, inhuman fiend. In the former situation he is portrayed as a totally normal individual who is simply a victim of circumstances; in the latter, as some less-than-human creature whose predatory attacks are his only sources of sexual gratification. Neither image corresponds to reality.

Perhaps this is as good a place as any to put to rest once and for all the myth that the rape victim is in any way responsible for the assault. Often it is argued in court that the victim has acted provocatively and seductively and, therefore, just got what she was "asking for." The dress, appearance, and behavior of the victim are in fact all beside the point. No matter how provocatively and invitingly the woman may have behaved—no matter if she was in fact a "tease"—"no" is "no." She can change her mind at any point she wants to. Now a man in that situation would understandably become frustrated and upset with her. He would most naturally become angry with her. He might swear at her and tell her off and have nothing more to do with her, but if he is well-adjusted, he will not rape her. There is no law against a wo-

[11] A. J. Davis, "Sexual Assaults in the Philadelphia Prison System and Sherriff's Vans," *Trans-action* 6, No. 2 (December 1968), pp. 8–16.
[12] Ibid., pp. 15–16.

man changing her mind at the very last moment, but there is a law against not respecting her right to do this.

In our many years of work with the sexual offender, however, we have yet to find a geniune case of sexual provocation on the part of the victim. This myth of a seducing and vindictive victim appears to be one of a number of misconceptions about rape that stem from the basic misunderstanding of rape as being motivated primarily by a need for sexual gratification. Other related myths include the idea that legalizing prostitution may help to reduce the incidence of rape. The incidence of rape is in fact alarming, and we know that most rapes go unreported, but legalizing prostitution will not help. Although not legal, prostitution does exist and is available as a sexual outlet to the rapist. But, in fact, it is not the case that the rapist rapes simply because he has no other sexual outlets. Many rapists are married or have regular sexual relationships with one or a number of women. When asked, "Why didn't you simply go to a prostitute instead of raping someone?" the offender usually replies "a real man never has to pay for it." We have seen, however, that what is motivating the rapist is not in fact a need for sexual gratification per se but that sex becomes a way of expressing other unresolved feelings and concerns. The idea that rape is the result of sexual desire is simplistic and inaccurate. Therefore, legalizing prostitution is no solution, nor is castration. This myth too reflects the simpleminded misconception of rape as the result of an "oversexed" individual or that basically it is a sexual urge that prompts rape. Likewise the belief that pornography contributes to rape is erroneous. All of these myths indicate a failure to realize that rape is in fact a complex, multidetermined act resulting from a large number of interrelated factors.

Often we are asked if there is anything a victim can do to avert a rape. Unfortunately, since rape is multidetermined, there is no sure thing a potential victim can do that will always successfully dissuade her would-be assailant. We have put the question to our patients themselves time and time again: "Was there ever anything an intended victim said or did that stopped you?" Their answers indicated that what works in one situation fails in another. For example, one rapist answered, "When my victim screamed, I ran;" another said, "When my victim screamed, I cut her throat."

SOME FACTS ABOUT THE RAPIST

The rapist is a complex human being and although there is a wide variety of individual differences among offenders who commit forcible and repetitive sexual assaults, there are a number of features that they share or have in common.

The most obvious fact is that the rapist is a *male*. Rape is a form of sexual deviation, and sexual deviation is far more characteristic of males than of females. There are many complex reasons for this—both psychological and sociological—but, to try to simplify the explanation, it appears that sexual deviation is symptomatic of conflicts in regard to a sense of identity. In the psychosocial development of the male it is more difficult to achieve a secure sense of identity than it is for the female. In part this is due to the absence of a clearly visible, concrete model for the male during formative years. In the course of development, the male and the female child have the mother as the principal identification and love object. It is the male who must relinquish this original love object and not become like mother (who is a visible, concrete image) but become like father (whose model is less visible, more abstract). The result is that the male is never as secure of his sense of identity in terms of being a man as the female is in terms of being a woman. The role definitions for the male are more artificial and he is denied some avenues of emotional expression permitted females; for example, when hurt or upset he is not expected to act hurt and his distress is characteristically transformed into anger or rage. Likewise such qualities as warmth, tenderness, and affection toward other males go undeveloped. It appears psychologically that there is a greater gap between what it is to be a "man" in our culture and what it is to be a human being than between what it is to be a "woman" and what it is to be a human being. The rapist is more likely to be a male, then, because the male is never as secure of his sense of identity as is the female. Furthermore, rape, as we have seen, is always in part an expression of anger and rage. When angered, a woman is more likely to withhold sexual relations. It is not considered degrading for a man to be "subjected" to sexual acts with a woman. Even in those rare cases where a man has been the victim of a sexual assault by a woman, the charges brought against the woman are likely to be "assault and battery" since the prosecution believes it would be next to impossible to convince a jury that a man had to be forced into a sexual act. Even where the victim is an under-aged person, the sexual involvement of an adult woman with an underaged male is seen as initiation, whereas the sexual involve-ment of an adult male with an underage female is seen as cor-ruption.

A second fact is that the rapist may be of any age. Though he is more likely to be a younger person, usually in his twenties, we have seen offenders ranging in age from early adolescence to late middle age. Some physical strength is needed to accomplish the as-sault, and when he reaches adulthood, the male then possesses suf-ficient strength to commit the offense. More important, however, it is at this age that the demands and responsibilities of adulthood are placed on the male; when psychologically unprepared to meet these demands, he decompensates under the impact of the result-ing stresses. The rape is in part a result of feeling overwhelmed by the pressures and the responsibilities of adulthood.

The rapist is of average intelligence. Offenders can be found in all levels of intellectual ability, but the majority—like the gen-eral population—fall within the average or normal range. Although he shows no significant defect in regard to intelligence, however, the educational and vocational achievement of the rapist appears to be much below his potential. It appears that his impulse-ridden behavior and inability to tolerate frustration interfere with his mastering the demands of school and of work successfully.

It is also typical that the rapist comes from the lower socio-economic levels of our society where there is little encouragement or opportunity to develop a sense of identity and masculinity through avenues other than sexuality and physical aggression. Emotional and psychological deprivation as well as social and economic limitations surround the disadvantaged individual. In the lower socioeconomic strata of our society, the occupant finds little or no opportunity to develop alternate means of dealing with frustration and disappointment; there is a greater absence of solid and stable identification figures (as a result, deep, consistent, and continuing parental love does not take place); model behavior ex-hibits a greater use of physical force for expression and for ef-forts at control; there are no agencies for socialization—an uncon-trolled setting encourages the development of an uncontrolled personality.

Rape as a Symptom

The act of forcible rape is in *every* instance symptomatic of psychological disturbance but it is not limited to any one specific diagnostic category. The finding of a basic neurotic structure is relatively rare, but the various types of personality disorders and more severe borderline and psychotic states are clearly represented. Most rapists, however, are neither psychotic nor mentally retarded, but they do appear to have in common certain general psychological characteristics that differentiate them from healthy, well-adjusted individuals.

Clinically, the most apparent features of the aggressive sexual offender are his defects in regard to impulse management, object (interpersonal) relations, and a sense of identity: This individual exhibits an inability to tolerate frustration and to delay impulse gratification. Instead, he discharges psychological stresses and tensions by acting out behaviorally rather than verbalizing his discomfort or gratifying his impulses through fantasy. His range of interests is narrow and shallow and he appears unable to pursue long-term, reality-oriented, goal-directed behavior. Instead, he is quickly overwhelmed by frustration and gives up easily in the face of failure. His impulse management is especially tenuous in regard to aggression. Either he tends to suppress his anger completely, never allowing any expression of it, or he is unable to control or modulate it at all—in neither case is he able to deal with his feelings in an appropriate and adaptive fashion. In the former situation he has no access to his own feelings; in the latter case his recognition of the demands of the external world is faulty.

This offender's defective interpersonal relationships suggest a marked developmental impairment in object relations. He is, by and large, socially insensitive and/or indifferent to the feelings and needs of others. Characteristically, he does not experience warmth and trust in his interpersonal relationships. He tends to see himself and his own needs as being the only fact of social relevance; other persons are regarded merely as obstacles to be overcome or as objects to be used for his own need gratification. Consequently, he has never been able to establish close, long-lasting relationships but instead could be regarded as a social isolate. His narcissistic, demanding orientation precludes any appreciation of the possibility of a mutual, reciprocal quality to a relationship. Instead, a cynical, self-centered, infantile value system operates, which, together with a system of projective defenses, works to exonerate the offender from a sense of personal responsibility (guilt) for his behavior and allows him to experience himself as the victim of an uncaring and hostile, even malevolent, world. The offender typically does not accept personal responsibility for his acts. He may deny that he did it or claim he cannot remember. Even when he does acknowledge his offense, there is usually much rationalization or minimization of the assault: "She really wanted it." "She looked older." "It only happened because I was drunk." He seems incapable of differentiating among others and tends to regard all human relationships in terms of using or being used. There are no feelings of attachment to other persons or even to possessions that are not eroticized or narcissistic. This quality of detachment results in a tendency to experience others as unreal, and such qualities as warmth, empathy, and trust are noticeably absent. He has never effected a close, meaningful, interpersonal relationship to anyone, male or female, in his life. In order to fend off the resultant sense of aloneness and emptiness, there is sometimes a peculiar alleged investment in abstractions such as courage, motherhood, or independence.

This individual seems not to be in touch with his own feelings. His general mood state is dysphoric, characterized by a dull depression; feelings of fear bordering on panic; anger, and irritation; and an overwhelming sense of purposelessness and hopelessness.

The dangerous sexual offender's defects in regard to his identity or sense of self are exhibited in the frustrations he experiences in his efforts to achieve an adequate masculine image, the stereotyped image he has of being a man, and the conflicts he meets in his desire to gain mastery over his life in active and assertive ways. Typically, there is a feeling of having failed to achieve a sense of confidence in himself as a man in both sexual and nonsexual areas—a feeling that is unacknowledged, for he exhibits little capacity for insight or self-observation. In fact, the extremes to which he goes to avoid facing himself suggest that deeply rooted feelings of emptiness, inadequacy, helplessness, insecurity, worthlessness, and vulnerability underlie his behavior. Consequently, aggressive sexuality comes to serve a compensatory function for perceived threats to his self-image. With increasing social failures in the social, academic, vocational, and marital sphere of his life, he is reduced to placing an ever increasing premium on sexuality and physical aggression for a sense of competency, mastery, and self-esteem—for a sense of being. His inability to manage personal responsibilities and to master life demands confronts him with the terror of being annihilated. Likewise, passivity, for the same reasons, is intolerable, and he has serious difficulty in dealing with any situation that places him in a passive position, such as relating to authority figures.

This tenuous sense of identity coupled with low self-esteem leads to aggressive acting-out often as a last resort against depression, self-destruction, and/or psychotic decompensation. Sexual assault, where aggression is the goal and sexuality the means, then becomes an effort at psychological survival; it becomes the offender's assertion of his existence and his potency; it becomes the denial of his vulnerability. Feelings of hurt and fear—"unmanly" emotions—are converted into anger and rage, which are more tolerable, more familiar, and more "masculine."

In some offenders these characteristics have been evident and pronounced from their early life and even though the rape may be their first sexual offense, it is but another expression of a pattern of chronic failure in managing life demands adaptively. In other offenders, these traits are less noticeable. These men appear to have succeeded in making some adequate life adjustment for the most part; however, their adjustment is tenuous, and under stress they decompensate and act-out. The rape here appears as an exception to what has been generally a life lived without repetitive conflict and difficulty with society and the law. Whether the act of rape is symptomatic of a long-standing and serious personality disorder or of a temporary regression under unusual stress, it is *always* symptomatic of some psychological defect.

THE ASSESSMENT OF SEXUAL DANGEROUSNESS

In order to determine whether or not a particular individual constitutes a danger to society, that is, in order to determine whether or not this person if released into the community is likely to commit a sexual assault that will jeopardize the physical safety of his victim, an intensive psychological study must be made of the offender and his offense. This includes a detailed examination of his background and early development; education, social and sexual development; military service; vocational history; marital status and relationship; medical and psychiatric history; and criminal record derived through clinical interviews, official records and transcripts, psychological tests, and field investigations. The estimation of the probability of future acting-out (sexual assault) then rests upon the clinician's skill, acumen, and expertise in evaluating these obtained data for their implications with reference to a number of issues.

1. Is the sexual offense primarily situational or symptomatic in nature? Does it stem for the most part from factors in the external world or from inner psychological dynamics of the offender? Is the offender a victim, an opportunist, or a predator?
2. What is the relationship between sexuality and aggression in the offense—is aggression in the service of sexual needs, sexuality in the service of aggressive needs, or are both a composite experience? Is the *modus operandi* one of seduction/enticement, threat/intimidation, or force/coercion? What motives underlie the offense? Why did the offense occur, and what is its meaning? What needs did it serve in the offender: dependent reaching out for object ties? retaliation or revenge? assertion or compensation (identity)? or narcissistic sexual gratification?
3. Where the offense is seen as symptomatic of psychological disturbance, how acute or chronic is this state? How early in the subject's development did behavior disturbance first begin to manifest itself? Does the offense constitute a fixation or a regression in the subject's psychosexual development?
4. What cognitive and emotional resources or skills does the subject possess to negotiate his interpersonal relationships and the demands of everyday life? What is the stability of his functioning? Is there any evidence of decompensation? Is he becoming progressively disorganized and unsuccessful in his ability to cope with the demands of reality?

The attempt, then, is to assess the individual's personality, his sense of identity, impulse management, object relations, and predominant affective states. When any of the following conditions are found to exist in the offender, the prognosis for dangerousness is ominous:

1. The faculties to understand and appreciate the consequences of his actions are impaired.
2. His abilities in regard to self-control are weakened or impaired or have never developed so that he cannot effect delay or management of his impulses.
3. He lacks empathetic identification with others, so although he understands, appreciates, and can make conscious decisions about his behavior, he simply does not care about the effect of his actions on others and is concerned only with himself.
4. Under certain life conditions (psychological stresses, alcoholic states, etc.) cognitive and perceptual distortions occur so that he misreads or misapprehends what is going on and cannot therefore respond appropriately.
5. Or, finally, he is a person who intends harm because injury to specified others becomes a source of gratification.

The dangerous sexual offender, then, jeopardizes the safety of his victim because he does not understand or appreciate the existing situation or, if he does, because he does not have the skill to manage it or, if he does, because he does not care to.

In the assessment of dangerousness, three major considerations must be taken into account: (1) the characterological features of the offender described above, (2) the emotional or psychological event lived out or expressed in the sexual assault (described in the section "Patterns of Rape"), and (3) the situational condition that elicited or supported such acts. In order to reach a decision in regard to the issue of dangerousness, the degree to which these factors continue to operate *both* in the *offender* and in the *environment* must be determined.

THERAPEUTIC MANAGEMENT
OF THE RAPIST

Rape is symptomatic of personal psychological developmental disability. To correct such a condition, then, a treatment program must approach the patient from all the directions of his life: physical, psychological, educational, spiritual, vocational, and social. What we are attempting to remedy, in essence, is human failure due basically to psychological immaturity. Therefore, the major objective of the program is to help the patient develop more effective methods of meeting and dealing with life demands.

Since we understand this patient's core defects to be rooted in his psychological development and expressed in his interpersonal relationship, psychotherapy is, in our view, the keystone in the arch of rehabilitation.

Our primary emphasis and major effort is to engage the patient in a therapeutic relationship that will permit him to work out his problems surrounding issues of identity, impulse management, and object relations. An individualized course of treatment is planned for each and every patient, taking into account his particular needs and resources. It is reviewed periodically and revised at any time it appears appropriate to do so. Both individual and group modes of therapy are provided, and generally each patient's treatment schedule involves a combination of both.

Since patients such as ours do not customarily seek out psychiatric treatment, there has been very little information available to us in the literature dealing with the treatment of sexually violent persons. Consequently, what we have learned has come about for the most part through search, exploration, trial and error, shared observations and discussions. What has emerged from our experiences to date is a number of considerations and issues that, although they may vary among our patients in regard to emphasis and importance, nevertheless seem to be rather inconsistent in their existence.

Facilities such as the Massachusetts Treatment Center offer the hope that aggressive, acting-out, sexual offenders can be treated and rehabilitated. In concept and implementation, it is an important departure from the way such individuals are customarily dealt with by our society. It is not a correctional institution that offers some therapy to its prisoners; it is a mental health facility designed to facilitate the amelioration of dangerous psychological defects in human beings. The following are factors of primary importance in its design.

Indefinite Confinement

An indeterminate period of segregation appears to be a necessary factor in the therapeutic management of a sexually dangerous person. The risk of further acting-out is too high for such a patient to be treated while in the community since different stages of effective treatment typically activate intense anxieties; Therefore, it is only on an inpatient basis that treatment should be attempted—it is analogous to quarantining a person with an infectious disease; it is necessary for his own protection as well as for the protection of others. Indefinite commitment serves a number of therapeutic aims. Whereas the sexual offender generally does not experience any felt need for treatment since he does not see himself as suffering from any psychological disorder, confinement motivates him toward treatment and places the responsibility for his rehabilitation squarely on his own shoulders—the choice is his: Free yourself of those problems that harm yourself and others and you will be free; remain as you are and you remain where you are. In addition, confinement initially removes a number of demands, responsibilities, and burdens from the patient—he does not have to work or support himself or his family; he does not have to structure his social activities; clothing, food, and housing are provided; etc.—thus freeing energies that can be deployed into treatment efforts. Finally, confinement appears to communicate a sense of external control—the patient feels protected from himself—and permits him to venture into the realm of self-examination and maturation.

Psychotherapy

Sexual offenses can be regarded as comparable to symptom formation; they constitute some type of attempt both to ward off intolerable feelings and to gratify unconscious wishes at the same time. They are *interpersonal* acts of psychogenic origin and, therefore, psychotherapy is regarded as the treatment of choice for the offender. It is in the interpersonal sphere that the offender's defects are most prominent and serious. Psychotherapy serves to remedy these defects where they exist: in the context of human interaction. Verbal interaction, communication with another human being permitted by the characteristic conditions of psychotherapy, offers an alternative to behavioral acting-out. Fellow human beings have been typically experienced by the offender as the course of his difficulties, problems, and suffering and consequently have become the object either of attack or of avoidance. Now in the guise of the therapist, a human being comes to be experienced as a source of assistance, comfort, and strength in helping the offender meet the emotional distresses and overcome the psychological handicaps of his life.

Specific therapy assignments are, of course, based on a thorough knowledge of the patient, his life experiences, his problems, and his resources; but in general we find that both group and individual psychotherapy are necessary modes of treatment. Group therapy orients the individual to his responsibilities to others and offers him the experience of being helped and cared for by others. The individual must function in the dual role of patient and therapist. He may take, but he is expected to also give—mutuality and reciprocity are underscored by the shared nature of a group. It is in the context of group especially that the individual may be directly confronted with the way he relates to others, the feelings he provokes in them toward him, the attempts he makes either to drive others away or to withdraw from others, etc., and it is in the group too that he may discover new ways of relating to others through invention, instruction, or example.

Individual psychotherapy permits the offender to uncover the derivatives of his experiences, to become more aware of the forces operating within him, to reexpose himself to the emotional experiences he could not handle adaptively, and to develop new and more appropriate ways of coping with them—in essence, to mature emotionally.

Psychotherapy constitutes the forum for the patient to reflect upon the underlying issues in the events and experiences that adversely affect his life and shape his behavior. Group therapy appears to elicit the difficulties the offender experiences in his peer relationship; whereas individual psychotherapy often seems to bring his difficulties in relating to authority figures into focus. Whatever the mode of therapy, however, a number of topics present themselves in the psychotherapy of the aggressive sexual offender that must be worked on and dealt with in order to remedy his psychopathology.

The initial phase of treatment is usually characterized by intense resistance on the part of the patient to acknowledging personal responsibility for both his criminal behavior (his symptoms) and his rehabilitation (his therapy). Typically, there is a tendency for the offender to deny or minimize or externalize responsibility for the offense (often projecting the responsibility of the assault onto the victim), to experience himself as the victim of external forces, and to regard others with wariness and distrust. A defensive anger (which may range in form and intensity from criticism and dissatisfaction with the adequacy and quality of hospital conditions and treatment services to outright belligerence, verbal abuse, and sometimes physical assault toward others) is expressed with emphasis placed more on "getting out" than on "getting well." Often there is pronounced antipathy toward authority figures who are seen as uncaring, punitive, nongiving, and abusive, which is especially directed toward the security (correctional) staff but also toward the mental health staff. In group sessions, fellow patients are regarded as incompetent, impotent, nonentities who will use whatever they learn about the individual to harass his life at the Center. Major difficulties are encountered in regard to the experience of ambivalent feelings toward others with the result that people are dichotomized into two mutually exclusive groups: the good (those "for" you—that is, those who agree with you) and the bad (those "against" you—that is, those who do not accept your deceptions). Faced with indefinite incarceration and with release contingent upon recovery, the offender's initial efforts at survival involve attempts to manipulate and exploit others, especially the therapist, through threat, intimidation, bribery, seduction, etc., and attempts to create divisiveness among those in charge (for example, between the mental health and the correctional staff or between the patient's therapist and other staff members, etc.) With proper handling, however, this pathological mode of relating (resistance) will prove ineffective and the fears and angers that characterize this initial phase of treatment can constitute the material by which the patient can become engaged in the treatment process and moved to the next phase of therapy in which the origins of his attitudes and perceptions of others become revealed.

In this uncovering phase, the dichotomies into which the offender places women (the virgin or the whore, the madonna or the bitch) and men (the tough guy or the weakling, the stud or the queer) can be seen to be derived from his relationship to his parents. The over-idealized (madonna) image of mother appears to be a reaction formation to mask the rage engendered by a mother who in fact was seductive, rejecting, suppressive, dominating, infantilizing, and narcissistic, but whose negative qualities were dealt with by being displaced onto substitute objects. Other women are seen as sexually promiscuous, castrating, and manipulating. Father generally was experienced as either cold, harsh, and brutal or as weak, impotent, and ineffectual and consequently was either hated, feared, scorned, and/or despised. In general, the patient felt controlled by mother and abandoned by father, instilling in him from a very early age a sense of helplessness and worthlessness.

The next level of therapeutic work is reached with the patient's experience and recognition of his own feelings of inadequacy and failure in meeting and mastering life demands, both sexual and nonsexual. Whereas initially he experienced himself as the victim of a malevolent world and next as the victim of unloving and negligent parents, he now comes to feel that he is a victim of himself and that he is in fact of no real worth (a message, incidentally, that a prison setting underlines and constantly reinforces). The patient's tenuous sense of identity becomes apparent in both sexual and nonsexual areas: He acknowledges heterosexual ignorance, incompetence, and confusion together with homosexual anxiety concerns and admissions of deviant interests such as exhibitionism and transvestism; in other areas there is a general sense of personal inadequacy (for example, he feels he is unintelligent) together with an extreme fear of passivity. While at one level passivity is terrifying to this patient for it represents a position of having no mastery over himself and his world and therefore jeopardizes his existence, at any other level it is deeply desired for it represents a position of literally being cared for. The dilemma of on the one hand wanting to turn over the responsibilities of his life management to others (since he feels incapable of self-mastery) and assume a passive-dependent position and on the other hand fearing that to do so would be tantamount to self-destruction since there is no one who would or could be capable, concerned, or caring enough to assume such responsibility (since he feels incapable of being loved) constitutes the core conflict operating within this type of patient. Essentially he experiences himself and his life as a succession of failures, especially in regard to engendering a response of interest, care, and love on the part of others toward him, and he sees himself as the reason for this: As others get to know me, they discover I am an unacceptable, unlikable person. Together with this negative self-image, low sense of personal worth, and insecure sense of identity, there exists a longing to be close to others, a sense of loss in this regard, and a concomitant feeling of depression. It is this combination of self-hatred, hurt, and depression that lies at the base of the sexual psychopathy. The rage, anger, and striking-out have all in part been measures to protect the patient from experiencing this intolerable depression and from destroying himself. In fact, frequently at this point in treatment suicidal thoughts and impulses appear.

Effective treatment depends on the therapist repeatedly communicating successfully in a variety of ways to the patient that he is neither abandoning him to his helplessness in mastering his life nor fostering such helplessness by assuming or accepting control over the patient's life and thereby depriving him of the opportunity to develop self-mastery. Instead the therapist communicates an attitude of confidence in the patient's ability to overcome his handicaps and of respect for him as a person of value and worth. When treatment is working, a number of issues generally become evident. Often the patient forms a deep attachment and loyalty to the therapist, often idealizing him and being jealous of his other patients and competing for his attention—this phase often has the character of an adolescent "crush." Frequently, the patient will take on the role of therapist or a quasi-parental role toward another patient whom he sees as "someone like he was once" and attempt to help him overcome his problems. The patient often comes to identify with the therapist both in regard to interests and values and typically expresses a desire to further his education and pursue some socially oriented profession such as teacher or counselor. Finally, there is a strong need to make restitution for his past behavior in part through the behaviors described above but also by attempting to contribute to the learning of others and by improving the lot of his fellow patients. Ultimately his goals become more realistic, he begins to pursue long-range activities, and he recognizes and is reasonably comfortable with his actual limitations. The most important clue to recovery, however, is the development of the ability to differentiate among others, to recognize that others have needs and feelings different and apart from his own, and to have regard and concern for the needs and feelings of others. Overall then, psychotherapy may be seen to progress through stages of resistance, uncovering, self-admission, restitution, and relearning. They are not separate and distinct phases but overlap and repeat. Unless each manifests itself and is fully dealt with, however, inpatient treatment cannot be considered complete.

Social Rehabilitation

In order for the patient to make use of psychiatric treatment, he cannot operate in a vacuum or in an environment of regimentation that does not recognize individual differences. Instead, a social system must be organized that will facilitate psychological development and maturation. Punishment has no place in such a system. Social infractions and unacceptable behavior are regarded as symptoms, and administration must work actively with the patient in order to understand what is motivating such behavior, what can be done to alleviate the distress, and how the patient can more adaptively manage such difficulties in the future. Responsibility on the part of the patient is emphasized, and in situations where actual damage has occurred, the patient is expected to repair it or to make reparation for it. Dispositions are always based on therapeutic considerations and the patient's therapist(s) may play an active role in such determinations. Treatment itself may, at times, be unpleasant or disagreeable but only incidentally—*never* intentionally.

In order to treat human failure effectively, medical, educational, vocational, recreational, and social programs are necessary to supplement and complement psychotherapy.

Although medical treatments (chemotherapy) are available, they should be underplayed and used very sparingly. It is the aim of mental health to orient the patient to people as sources of relief from distress and to have human beings psychologically replace the patient's dependency on nonhuman sources of pain relief (alcohol, drugs, etc.). Good health habits must be taught, however, and qualified medical attention must be given to the physical problems of the patient.

Effective educational and vocational programs help the pateient to overcome handicaps and to develop skills and abilities that will help him adapt more successfully to the world. Religious counseling for those to whom such is important can often facilitate self-respect and concern for others as well as alleviating a sense of isolation and worthlessness. Recreational programs can develop physical skills and a sense of interdependency with others, as well as affording health outlets for tension relief. Social programs are essential for helping the patient to develop social skills and to feel in contact with the outside world. Especially effective in this regard has been the participation of a number of senior college women who have worked as volunteers in conjunction with a seminar in clinical psychology conducted by one of us (A.N.G.). Functioning as paraclinicians under the supervision of the interdisciplinary clinical staff, these women work with selected patients toward the goals of resocialization. The contexts of their participation have included such programs as drama groups, music groups, tutoring, speech therapy, and art therapy as well as individual and group sociotherapy meetings. Other socialization programs include hobby clubs, a chapter of Alcoholics Anonymous, and a local Jaycee chapter. Not only do these programs contribute directly to the rehabilitation of the offender but also they often provide the context for issues that the patient then brings into his psychotherapy sessions.

Graduated Release

Hopefully, the patient will again face the responsibilities of freedom, and in order to facilitate this goal there needs to be a program of graduated responsibility and privilege. The transition to the community is facilitated by day care, night care, work release, educational release, temporary leave, and halfway house programs. Again the emphasis on psychotherapy remains and the patient continues to work with his assigned therapist(s) until it is very clear that he is no longer in need of such assistance. Five years appears to be a minimum estimate of outpatient treatment in our experience.[13]

In summary, the therapeutic management of sexually dangerous persons operates on the philosophy that sexual assaults can be understood as corresponding to symptom formation: They represent psychological defects and constitute some type of attempt by the offender to ward off intolerable intrapsychic experiences. To remedy such a condition the individual must be given psychological treatment in a setting that encourages maturation and rehabilitation. He must be dealt with as a patient, not a

---

[13]The average treatment schedule for our patients is one hour of individual psychotherapy and two hours of group psychotherapy each week.

prisoner. He must be confined to a mental health facility, not a prison. Treatment, not punishment, is the only avenue to the restoration of health in the offender and safety in the society. Furthermore, only through careful study and research afforded in such a facility will clinicians advance their knowledge of treating these offenders and ultimately progress toward identification of early warning symptoms. A maximum security mental health facility is a meaningful alternative to a correctional institution in rehabilitating repetitive, dangerous, aggressive, antisocial offenders.

It is our belief[14] that morality and law make preventive detention justifiable only when treatment is available and adequate—preventive detention is then preventive medicine. Effectiveness of treatment is a goal and not a requirement, a goal that we feel can only be realized when there is opportunity to apply established methods and to explore, with proper safeguards, new methods.

The clinician in his role as described here is not concerned with the mental health model of primary or even secondary prevention. Regardless of the social, political, and economic factors that so distorted, disrupted, or destroyed an individual's socialization, his sexual and aggressive impulses, or his discharge and control apparatus; and without consideration of the terrible inequities of our social and economic system that restricts and constrains the available resources for socially acceptable emotional and personal expression of the poor and the oppressed; and, further, without regard for the conflicting sexual and aggressive attitudes of our society and its leaders that enhance conflicts and create mental confusion, some individuals under certain conditions have a high probability of committing a violent sexual assault. It is the clinician's task to bring to bear whatever his science, his theories, and his experience teach him to assist society in identifying and treating such persons.

It is apparent from our previous remarks that we fully recognize the inadequacies of this science in the prediction of dangerousness and in the treatment of the offenders so diagnosed. It should also be apparent that despite this we believe that society has a responsibility to protect its members from unwarranted violence and has the right to use preventive detention as one protec-

---

[14] M. L. Cohen, A. N. Groth and R. Siegel, "The Clinician's Approach to Dangerousness and Social Policy Issues," unpublished paper presented to the American Psychological Association, September 1974.

tive procedure. Society, however, also has obligations to the individual who may be subject to such a procedure and with regard to this we offer the following:

1. At least with respect to the sexually dangerous person, special, separate centers for his commitment and treatment should exist.
2. Treatment facilities should be such in fact and not only in name. We are all aware that with rare exceptions the treatment personnel in most correctional or special care units are poorly trained, are inadequately supervised, and have no active teaching or training program available to increase their skills.
3. Rigorous safeguards should be provided for periodic review of persons committed under such laws—a minimum of yearly reviews in addition to reviews initiated by the offender.
4. Since such laws are involved in behavioral prediction, behavioral scientists and clinicians other than psychiatrists should be designated as having advisory roles for the court. Such clinicians and scientists called upon to give expert testimony should be required to receive training in those aspects of the law relevant to criminal and mental health statutes.
6. In a like manner, separate courts should be established where the court personnel have had special training in the behavioral sciences.

Lastly, it is clear to us that the clinician or behavioral scientist must restrict his direct testimony to the predictive probabilities and the conditions of its limits. No clinician should be given, nor should he attempt to usurp, the right of society to determine the risks it is willing to take in the conflict between the safety of its members and the restrictions of a person's liberty. That decision is a political–social decision to be made by the selected representatives of society.

13

the sexually abused

The past several years have seen an increase in the awareness of and sensitivity to the problem of sexual violence in this country. Emergency rooms are establishing protocol for the management of the sexually abused person at the time of entry into the health care system, mental health services are providing follow-up counseling for the victim, and victims themselves are feeling freer to report the crime when it happens so that they may receive proper health care.

This chapter reports on a counseling and research study of victims of sexual assault seen at a large urban city hospital.[1] Over a 2-year period, over 300 cases were analyzed and three diagnostic categories were defined: rape trauma, accessory-to-sex, and sex-stress situation. These categories and suggested models of treatment are presented here as guidelines for clinicians to use in their work with victims of sexual assault both in the hospital and in the community setting.

[1] A. W. Burgess and L. L. Holmstrom, *Rape: Victims of Crisis* (Bowie, Md.: Robert J. Brady Company, 1974)

RAPE TRAUMA SYNDROME

Rape trauma syndrome[2] is the acute phase and long-term reorganization process that occurs as a result of forcible rape or attempted forcible rape. This syndrome of behavioral, somatic, and psychological reactions is an acute stress reaction to a life-threatening situation.

Rape traume syndrome is usually a two-phase reaction. The first is the acute phase. This is the period in which there is a great deal of disorganization in the victim's life-style as a result of the rape. Physical symptoms are especially noticeable, and one prominent feeling noted is fear. The second phase begins when the victim begins to reorganize the life-style. Although the time of onset varies from victim to victim, the second phase often begins about 2 to 3 weeks after the attack. Motor activity changes, and nightmares and phobias are especially likely during this phase.

The medical regimen for the rape victim involves the prescription of antipregnancy and antivenereal disease medication after the physical and gynecological examination. The procedure often includes prescribing 25 to 50 mg of diethylstilbesterol a day for 5 days to protect against pregnancy and 4.8 million units of aqueous procaine penicillin intramuscularly to protect against venereal disease. Symptoms reported by the victim need to be distinguished as either side effects of the medication or as conditions resulting from the sexual assault.

The Acute Phase: Disorganization

Impact reactions. In the immediate hours following the rape, the victim may experience an extremely wide range of emotions. The impact of the rape may be so severe that feelings of shock or disbelief are expressed. When interviewed within a few hours of the rape, the victims in this study mainly showed two emotional styles:[3] the expressed style, in which feelings of fear, anger, and anxiety were shown through such behavior as crying, sobbing, smiling, restlessness, and tenseness, and the controlled style in

[2] Sections reprinted with permission from A. W. Burgess and L. L Holmstrom, "Rape Trauma Syndrome," *Amer. J. Psychiatry* 131, No. 9 (September 1974), 981–86. Copyright 1974 by the American Psychiatric Association.

[3] A. W. Burgess and L. L. Holmstrom, "The Rape Victim in the Emergency Ward," *Amer. J. Nursing* 73, No. 10 (October 1973), 1741-1745.

which feelings were masked or hidden and a calm, composed, or subdued affect was seen. A fairly equal number of victims showed each style.

Somatic reactions. During the first several weeks following a rape, many of the acute somatic manifestations described below are evident.

1. *Physical trauma.* This includes general soreness and bruising from the physical attack in various parts of the body such as the throat, neck, breasts, thighs, legs, and arms. Irritation and trauma to the throat were especially a problem for those women forced to have oral sex.
2. *Skeletal muscle tension.* Tension headaches and fatigue as well as sleep pattern disturbances were common symptoms. Victims were either not able to sleep or would fall asleep only to wake and not be able to go back to sleep. Victims who had been suddenly awakened from sleep by the assailant frequently found that they would wake each night at the time the attack had occurred. The victim might cry or scream out in her sleep. Victims also described experiencing a startle reaction—they become edgy and jumpy over minor incidents.
3. *Gastrointestinal irritability.* Victims might complain of stomach pains. The appetite might be affected and the victim might state that she is not eating, the food has no taste, or she feels nauseated from the antipregnancy medication. Victims also report feeling nauseated just thinking of the rape.
4. *Genitourinary disturbance.* Gynecological symptoms such as vaginal discharge, itching, a burning sensation on urination, and generalized pain were common. A number of women developed chronic vaginal infections following the rape. Rectal bleeding and pain were reported by victims who had been forced to have anal sex.

Emotional reactions. Victims express a wide gamut of feelings as they begin to deal with the aftereffects of the rape. These feelings range from fear, humiliation, and embarrassment to anger, revenge, and self-blame. Fear of physical violence and death was the primary feeling described. Victims stated that it was not the rape that was so upsetting as much as the feeling that they would be killed as a result of the assault. One woman stated: "I am really mad. My life is disrupted; every part of it is upset. And I have to be grateful I wasn't killed. I thought he would murder me."

Self-blame was another reaction women described partly because of their socialization to the attitude of "blame the victim." For example, one young woman had entered her apartment building one afternoon after shopping. As she stopped to take her keys from her purse, she was assaulted in the hallway by a man who then forced his way into her apartment. She fought him to the point of taking a knife and using it against him and in the process she was quite severely beaten, bruised, and raped. Later she said

> I keep wondering maybe if I had done something different when I first saw him that it wouldn't have happened—neither he nor I would be in trouble. Maybe it was my fault. See, that's where I get when I think about it. My father always said whatever a man did to a woman, she provoked it.

The Long-Term Process: Reorganization

All victims in the subsample group of rape trauma experienced some degree of disorganization in their life-style; their presence at the emergency room of the hospital was testimony to that fact. Various factors affected their coping behavior to the trauma, i.e., ego strength, social network support, and the way people treated them as victims. This coping and reorganization process began at different times for the individual victims.

Motor activity. The long-term effects of the rape generally consisted of an increase in motor activity, especially through changing residence. The move, in order to ensure safety and to facilitate the victim's ability to function in a normal style, was very common. Many victims changed residence within a relatively short period of time after the rape. There was also a strong need to get away, and some women took trips even to other states or countries.

Changing one's telephone number was a common reaction. It was often changed to an unlisted number. The victim might do this as a precautionary measure or as the result of threatening or obscene telephone calls. The victim was haunted by the fear that the assailant knew where she was and would come back for her.

Another common response was to turn for support to family members not normally seen daily. In most cases the victim told her parents what had happened but occasionally the victim contacted her parents for support and did not explain why she was suddenly interested in talking with them or being with them.

Nightmares. Dreams and nightmares could be very upsetting and many victims, during follow-up conversations, spontaneously described very frightening dreams, as illustrated in the following.

> I had a terrifying nightmare and shook for 2 days. I was at work and there was this maniac killer in the store. He killed two of the salesgirls by slitting their throats. I'd gone to set the time clock and when I came back the two girls were dead. I thought I was next. I had to go home. On the way I ran into two girls I knew. We were walking along and we ran into the maniac killer and he was the man who attacked me—he looked like the man. One of the girls held back and said, "No—I'm staying here." I said I knew him and was going to fight him. At this point I woke with the terrible fear of impending doom and fright. I knew the knife part was real because it was the same knife the man held to my throat.

Victims report two types of dreams. One is similar to the example above where the victim wishes to do something but then wakes before acting. As time progresses, the second type may occur: The dream material changes somewhat, and frequently the victim reports mastery in the dream—being able to fight off the assailant. A young woman reported the following dream a month after being raped.

> I had a knife and I was with the guy and I went to stab him and the knife bent. I did it again and he started bleeding and he died. Then I walked away laughing with the knife in my hand.

This dream woke up the victim; she was crying so hard that her mother came in to see what was wrong. The girl stated that in her waking hours she never cries.

Phobic reactions. The development of phobic reactions is a common phenomenon, which occurs as a defensive reaction to the circumstances of the rape. The following are the most common phobic reactions among victims in the sample.

Fear of indoors. This occurred in victims who had been attacked while sleeping in their beds. As one victim said, "I feel better outside. I can see what is coming. I feel trapped inside. My fear is of being inside, not outside."

Fear of outdoors. This occurred in victims who had been attacked outside their homes. These women felt safe inside but would walk outside only with the protection of another person or only when necessary. As one victim stated, "It is sheer terror for every step I take. I can't wait to get to the safety of my own place."

Fear of being alone. Almost all victims reported fears of being alone after the rape. Often the victim had been attacked when alone, when no one could come to her rescue. One victim said, "I can't stand being alone. I hear every little noise—the windows creaking. I am a bundle of nerves."

Fear of crowds. Many victims were quite apprehensive when they had to be in crowds or ride on public transportation. One 41-year-old victim said,

> I'm still nervous from this, when people come too close—like when I have to go through the trolley station and the crowds are bad. When I am in crowds I get the bad thoughts. I will look over at a guy and if he looks really weird, I hope something bad will happen to him.

Fear of people behind them. Some victims reported fear of people walking behind them. This was often common if the victim had been approached suddenly from the rear. One victim said,

> I can't stand to have someone behind me. When I feel someone is behind me, my heart starts pounding. Last week I turned on a guy that was walking in back of me and waited till he walked by. I just couldn't stand it.

Sexual fears. Many women experience a crisis in their sexual life as a result of the rape. Their normal sexual style has been disrupted. For the women who had no prior sexual activity, the incident was especially upsetting since they had nothing to compare the experience with to know that normal sexual activity is not as they experienced it. For the women who were sexually active, their fear increased when they were confronted by their husband or boyfriend to resume sexual relations. One victim said,

> My boyfriend thought the rape might give me a negative feeling to sex and he wanted to be sure it didn't. That night as soon as we were back to the apartment he wanted to make love. I didn't want sex, especially that night . . . . He also admitted he wanted to know if he could make love to me or if he would be repulsed by me and unable to.

This victim and her boyfriend had considerable difficulty resuming many aspects of their relationship besides the sexual part. Many women were unable to resume a normal sexual style during the acute phase and persisted with the difficulty. One victim reported, 5 months after the assault, "There are times I get hysterical with my boyfriend. I don't want him near me. I get panicked. Sex is okay, but I still feel like screaming."

Management of Rape Trauma Syndrome

There are several basic assumptions underlying the model of crisis intervention to be used in counseling the rape victim.

1. The rape represents a crisis in that the victim's life-style may be disrupted physically, psychologically, socially, and sexually.
2. The victim is regarded as a "normal" person who is functioning adequately prior to the crisis situation.
3. Crisis counseling is the treatment model of choice to return the victim to the previous level of functioning as quickly as possible. The crisis counseling is issue-oriented intervention. Previous problems are not considered a priority for discussion; in no way is the counseling considered psychotherapy. When other issues of major concern were identified that indicated another treatment model, referrals should be offered if the victim so requests them.
4. The counselor takes the active role in initiating therapeutic contact as opposed to more traditional methods where the patient is expected to be the initiator.

Management of Compounded Reaction

There will be some rape victims who have either past or current history of physical, psychiatric, or social difficulties along with the rape trauma syndrome. It usually becomes quite clear that these people need more than crisis counseling. When rape victims are known to other therapists, physicians, or agencies, it is suggested that the counselor assume a secondary position. Support should be provided for the rape experience, especially if the victim presses charges and goes through the court process, but the counselor can work in a secondary position with the primary agency or therapist. It is not unusual to note that victims with compounded reactions develop additional symptoms such as depression, psychotic behavior, psychosomatic disorders, suicidal behavior, and acting-out behavior associated with alcoholism, drug use, and sexual activity.

Management of Silent Rape Reaction

Since a significant proportion of victims still not not report a rape, counselors should be alert to a syndrome that is called the *silent reaction to rape.* This reaction occurs in the victim who has not told anyone of the rape, who has not settled her feelings and reactions on the issue, and who is carrying a tremendous psychological burden.

Evidence of such a syndrome became evident as a result of collecting life history data from the sample of rape victims. A number of women stated that they had been raped or molested at a previous time, often when they were children or adolescents. Often these women had not told anyone of the rape and had just kept the burden within themselves. The current rape reactivated their reaction to the prior experience. It became clear that because they had not talked about the previous rape, the syndrome continued to develop and these women had carried unresolved issues with them for years. They would talk as much of the previous rape as they did of the current rape.

A diagnosis of this syndrome should be considered when the counselor observes any of the following symptoms during an assessment interview.

1. Increasing signs of anxiety as the interview progresses, such as long periods of silence, blocking of associations, minor stuttering, and physical distress.
2. The patient reports sudden marked irritability or actual avoidance of relationships with men or marked change in sexual behavior.
3. History of sudden onset of phobic reactions and fear of being alone, going outside, or being inside alone.
4. Persistent loss of self-confidence and self-esteem, an attitude of self-blame, paranoid feelings, or dreams of violence and/or nightmares.

Counselors who suspect that the patient was raped in the past should be sure to include questions concerning the woman's sexual behavior in the evaluation interview and to ask if anyone has ever attempted to assault her. Such questions may release considerable pent-up material relevant to forced sexual activity.

Discussion

The crisis that results when a victim has been sexually assaulted is in the service of self-preservation. The victim generally believes that living is better than dying and that was the choice that had to be made. The victims' reactions to the impending threat to their lives is the nucleus around which an adaptive pattern may be noted.

The coping behavior of individuals to life-threatening situations has been noted in the work of such writers as Grinker and Spiegel,[4] Lindemann,[5] Kubler-Ross,[6] and Hamburg.[7] Kubler-Ross wrote of the process patients go through to come to terms with the fact of dying. Hamburg wrote of the resourcefulness of patients in facing catastrophic news and discussed a variety of implicit strategies by which patients face threats to life. This broad sequence of the acute phase, group support, and the long-run resolution described by these authors is compatible with the psychological work rape victims must do over time.

The majority of rape victims will be able to reorganize their life-style after the acute symptom phase, stay alert to possible threats to their life-style, and focus upon protecting themselves from further insult if they have some type of crisis intervention.

ACCESSORY-TO-SEX SYNDROME

This second diagnostic category describes a group of sexual trauma victims—primarily children and adolescents—called *accessory-to-sex victims.*[8] In this type of sexual situation, victims are pressured into sexual activity by a person who stands in a power position over them as through age, authority, or some other way. This victim is unable to consent either because of personality or cognitive development. The emotional reaction of victims result from their being pressured into sexual activity and from the added tension of keeping the act secret.

Accessory-to-sex cases may be categorized according to whether the incident occurs once, several times within a short period of time, or over an extended time period of months or

[4] Roy R. Grinker and John P. Spiegel, *Men Under Stress* (Philadelphia: Blakiston, 1945).

[5] Eric Lindemann, "Symptomotology and Management of Acute Grief," *American Journal of Psychiatry* **101** (1944), 141–148.

[6] Elizabeth Kubler-Ross, "On Death and Dying," *Journal of American Medical Association* **221** (1972), 174–179.

[7] David Hamburg, "A Perspective on Coping Behavior," *Archives of General Psychiatry* **17** (1967), 277–284.

[8] Sections reprinted with permission from Ann W. Burgess and Lynda L. Holmstrom, "Sexual Trauma of Children and Adolescents: Pressure, Sex, and Secrecy," *Nursing Clinics of North America* **10** (3) Sept. 1975: 551–63. Copyright 1975 by W. B. Saunders Company.

years. There also may be attempted accessory-to-sex cases in which the offender attempts to pressure the child but the child escapes the sexual activity.

Frequently the offender is a family member such as father, stepfather, grandfather, uncle, or cousin. These people have re-peated access to the child because they are a family member and their presence is not questioned by the family.

Pressurizing the Victim into Sexual Activity

The offender stands in a relationship of dominance to the victim. Ambivalence as a component of the decision-making proc-ess is characteristic of the young person's emotional life and the offender trades on this. Georg Simmel, in discussing domination as a form of interaction, states that the desire for domination is aimed to break the internal resistance of the subordinate.[9]

In accessory to sex, the offender pressures the victim into being an accessory to the sexual activity, that is, to go along with it at least once. The victim may be totally unaware that sexual activity is part of the offer. One victim described her happy visits to her grandparents' farm and how she enjoyed being thrown into the haystack. One day her grandfather said he would throw her into the haystack and give her a silver dollar if she did something with him. The child went along with him assuming it would be fun as she had previously experienced, but it turned out very differently.

As in this example, some method of pressure or offer is made to the person—i.e., being thrown into the haystack and money. Three main types of pressure are used by the offenders.

Material goods. Children are most likely to be offered some type of material goods such as candy or money. In one case in-volving a 6-year-old girl and her 6-year-old male cousin, the girl said

> Big Bobby asked me and Joey to come to see his puppies. Then he said he'd give us some money to take down our pants.

The situation advanced to where the girl was further pressured into sexual activity and penetration was attempted by the of-fender.

[9]Kurt H. Wolff, *The Sociology of Georg Simmel* (London: The Free Press of Glencoe, 1950), p. 181.

Misrepresenting moral standards. Family members can pressure the child by telling the child it is "okay to do." As one victim said, "If an adult tells you to do something, you do it." In the case of a 5-year-old, a neighbor offender pressured the child into "playing house" with him. The matter came to the attention of the mother when she discovered blood on her child's pants.

Young people often do not have the ability to consent when confronted with pressure of material goods or when an adult misrepresents moral standards. Children under age six and latency-age children may know that sexual situations between themselves and adults are wrong but their total concept of sexuality has not incorporated into their life-style and they go along with the pressure from the adult in the situation. The following example illustrates this inability to make a decision until it was too late.

> He made me lie down . . . and then he showed me his penis and I remember him talking to me and telling me he was going to put that inside of me and he showed me where he was going to put it and he made me touch my vagina and he made me touch his penis. That's when I decided that there was no way—I looked at this thing and I looked at me and thought no way. And I got upset and I tried to get away from him but he said, "Oh, I'm going to throw you in the haystack; everything will be all right, everything will be okay." And he kept telling me that. Then he started to enter me and I can just remember the pain . . . .

Need for human contact. The majority of accessory-to-sex victims are children and adolescents; however, the victim sample also did include some adult women who did not have the cognitive or emotional development to be able to consent or not to consent. These women were extremely isolated and impoverished socially and emotionally and they were enticed by men by their need for human warmth and contact.

Physical Reaction to the Sexual Activity

The type of sexual activity that the offender attempted to achieve ranged from approaching the victim and pressure (attempted) to full sexual penetration of the victim. Hand to genital contact as well as mouth to genital contact might also have been part of the activity.

Children usually described the experience in terms of whether it hurt, a negative reaction, or whether it was pleasurable, a positive reaction. More often than not, the child experiences a negative reaction and sometimes this reaction serves to disrupt the offender's intent and he leaves the scene as in the following case.

> A 6-year-old girl stated that a man followed her into her building and offered her a bag of candy. She said, "He took me inside the hall and put his hands in my pants and pinched me and I cried." The man left the scene at that point and the child ran to tell her mother. The mother noted blood on the child's pants, notified the police, and brought the child to the hospital.

There are some victims who find the sexual activity pleasurable. Such situations tend to be the cases where hand–genital contact is used rather than penetration. One 19-year-old recounting her childhood experiences with her grandfather said,

> He would sit me in his lap with my legs slightly spread apart and stroke my inner thighs, labia, and genital area . . . . I found it very pleasurable. I would have my back against his torso, my head on his chest and sometimes fall asleep. He was always so warm and gentle and he would tell me stories.

Pressured into Secrecy

If the offender is successful with his victim, he must now try to conceal the deviate behavior from others. More likely than not, he will try to pledge the victim to secrecy in several ways. The child may not necessarily be aware of the existence of the secret as in situations in which the act is gentle and pleasurable and the child does not believe it is wrong. The offender may say this is something secret between them or, in some cases, he may threaten harm to the child if she does tell.

In most situations, however, the burden of the pressure to keep the secret is psychologically experienced as fear. Victims have spontaneously described the following fears, which they said bound them to the secret.

Fear of punishment. The victim often fears punishment if she tells. As one victim said,

> I don't remember anything wrong with it till Dad began to threaten me if I told . . . . There was pressure to go along with him. . . . He said he would punish me if I told mother.

Fear of repercussions from telling. Some victims do not think they would be believed. As one 23-year-old victim said in reflecting back on why she did not tell her parents, "You know to this day I don't think they (parents) would have believed me."

Some victims never tell because they fear the rejection the outside person will have to the disclosure. One victim said her parents "never would have acted right." Or the child may fear being blamed for the activity. One victim said,

> I think I never told because father (offender) might have said I was lying or I was a bad child and no one would like me again.

In two separate situations, the children were blamed after the disclosure. One 19-year-old victim (male) said, "Mother made us feel we were the cause of her brother being bad and wouldn't let us talk to our cousins."

Fear of abandonment or rejection. Children may fear that revealing the secret will cause catastrophic results. As one victim said,

> I thought it would be terrible to be separated from the family. I thought something terrible would happen if I told . . . . . The fear of rejection was really great as a child.

Communication barrier. Children do have difficulty sometimes putting a description of the activity into words and often times the child tells another companion who, in turn, tells an outside person. Children may not know the adult words. One victim describes this:

> . . . that's extremely rare when a kid would really be able to waltz up to Mom and say, "Guess what? Guess what your father did to me? Is it wrong for Grandpa to stick his thing into me?" I mean, can you just imagine?

Disclosure of the Secret

In many situations, the secret is broken within a certain time period. A secret disclosed without both parties' consent may be termed *betrayal*. Thus, there is the ever present tension that the secret may be betrayed. Simmel describes a "secret being surrounded by temptation and possibility of betrayal; and the external danger of being discovered is interwoven with the internal danger . . . of giving oneself away."[10]

The disclosure of the activity becomes a key clinical factor. The emotional reaction of the victim is greatly influenced by how and when the secret is disclosed and the resulting behavior from the outside person. There are several ways in which the secret may be disclosed.

Direct confrontation. There are times when the act will be observed by others and direct confrontation will occur. In the case of a 12-year-old mentally retarded girl who was seen being led into a neighbor's house, the police were notified. Upon entering the room of the man, they found the offender in the act of intercourse with the girl. Or there are situations in which the child is confronted with the fact that someone has found out about the sexual activity. One 19-year-old woman recounts her childhood experience in which her mother confronted her as follows:

> One time when I came back from a weekend with my grandparents, my mother wouldn't talk to me . . . she finally said she was disgusted with me and that she knew what my grandfather and I were doing and that I would have to tell a priest in confession . . . . I knew what she meant because no one else did what he did . . . . She wouldn't talk to me for days and I was upset and mad at her. It was her father and he told me to and I was supposed to obey elders and I didn't think it was wrong. So why was she mad at me? Why wasn't she mad at him?

Victim tells someone. Some victims were able to tell a parent or outside person directly about the sexual activity. For example, one 9-year-old was able to tell her mother that her stepfather had been "fooling" with her.

The clue. Visible clues were provided by many victims who were unable to tell someone directly. These clues included children walking home without any clothes on, children staying out all night, and pregnancy. The more subtle clues were the mother noticing an accumulation of nickels and dimes or new clothes. Another mother asked why the children were eating lollipops all the time and was told, "Uncle Jimmy gave it to me and told me not to tell you." Or the child may draw a picture or write a note. One mother told how she discovered the situation.

[10] Ibid., p. 334.

My daughter half hinted at it and I had a funny feeling something was wrong so I pumped her. We were sitting at the table having coffee and my husband asked her to do something and she said no. I asked her to do something and she did it. Later she asked me if I knew why she did things for me and not for my husband. I said no. And she said she would tell me some other time—it was grown-up stuff. Well, I got this awful feeling and I knew I had to find out so I asked her. She said she couldn't tell me but would draw it . . . . I took one look at what she drew on the paper and I went kookey.

Signs and symptoms. If the sexual activity continues over tim, signs and symptoms often develop and these may be brought to the attention of a professional.

Some parents observe the signs such as the child staying inside more frequently, not wanting to go to school, crying with no provocation, taking excessive number of baths, or a sudden onset of bedwetting and they become suspicious and seek professional help. The following illustrates this.

The mother of a 15-year-old girl stated to the nurse, "Mary is taking baths constantly and keeps complaining of stomachaches. She gets very upset when one of our neighbors comes around. She used to like going riding with him and he took her for cokes and donuts . . . . I am suspicious of what might be going on.

It was learned that the 35-year-old neighbor man had been pressuring the girl into sexual activity and this was producing the somatic and behavioral symptoms.

A variety of symptoms may be described by the child and the parent or the professional decodes the message. The symptoms may be gastrointestinal where the child vomits or complains of stomachaches, the development of a urinary tract infection, or the development of a medical condition such as pneumonia or mononucleosis. The following case illustrates how a silent reaction was missed during the first hospitalization but picked up the next time by the mother and the nurse and physician.

An 11-year-old girl was admitted with 2-day history of right lower quadrant pain, which is absent now; sharp and intermittent without exaccerbation or worsening over a 2-day period; no vomiting or diarrhea. Sore throat for 1 day. No other remarkable findings except that 1 year ago she was admitted to another hospital with similar pain and was hospitalized for 5 days and diagnosed to have pelvic inflammation.

A careful history obtained from the patient and her mother separately revealed the following:

Patient told mother last evening that she was sexually assaulted by her father four times. Parents are now separated and divorce proceedings in progress. The child states that 6 months ago she and her four siblings were staying alone with their father (mother had left the house for 4 weeks following parental argument). Father would either put the other children to bed early or send them on errands and then tell the child to go to his bed. She would do so. He would then tell her to pull down her pants and he would do likewise. He would put "vaseline on his pickle" and would "put it into her." She thought it went "into her bum." She did not look, turned her head, and screamed. She was lying on her back each time. This scene happened two times previously approximately 1 year ago when her mother was absent from the home. The patient told her two siblings that her father told her that if she told anyone he would kill her so she never told her mother until last evening. The mother was questioning her about the ordinary games played when she stayed with her father and the patient then related the "dirty game" story. Mother became disturbed and brought the child to the clinic and wants to press charges against her husband.

Management of the Victim

There are several important areas the clinician should be alert to in diagnosing and intervening with the accessory-to-sex victim.

Encouraging the child to talk. Many of the children spontaneously talked about the incident although the family might find it difficult to discuss. The parents need to talk about how they are encouraging or discouraging the child to talk about it. One mother said, "She talks about it. I tell her to forget it. She gets nervous when his name is mentioned." In another situation a mother said

She has brought it up three times today. I try to ignore it so she won't think about it but she keeps talking about it.

In this situation, the mother was encouraged to talk about her feelings and told it was a normal sign for the girl to talk about it and that when she had talked enough about it she would probably stop. And she did.

Draw-a-picture. Some children will return for clinic visits as part of the treatment regimen. The method of drawing pictures of what happened as a method to ensure the child was settling the experience was discovered in working with two sisters, ages 9 and 10, who had been molested by their stepfather. The sisters had seen the hospital psychiatrist and later said to a victim counselor

> I was afraid he was going to ask me to draw a picture of what happened but he didn't . . . .

Further in the conversation one sister said, "I know what he was trying to get me to say. He was a psychiatrist and wanted to know my reaction." The sisters were quite agreeable to using crayons to draw the scene, which included two stick figures lying side-by-side in bed. This prompted further discussion of the actual details of the activity and the children were quite intent to talk about the details they had drawn on the paper. Encouraging children to talk about their experiences is an open and healthy way to deal with the tensions that have built over the secrecy process.

Observing symptoms over time. Parents need to be instructed about the possible physical and behavioral symptoms that can develop in the child from the pressure of the situation and that are considered within the normal range for this reaction to a stress situation.

Minor phobic symptoms may be reported when the victim sees or hears the offender's name or sees him. One 12-year-old mentally retarded girl who was unable to verbalize her concerns would run into the house whenever she would see the offender in the neighborhood. Another victim described her change in behavior:

> . . . afterwards I just wanted to get away from him. I was afraid to go where he was after that. Didn't like visiting there anymore in the summer. I stayed in the house a lot . . . used the chamber pot under the bed rather than using the bathroom.

Changes in sleep patterns may be noted as well as the occurrence of dreams and nightmares. One victim described a recurrent dream that she had around the age of 7 or 8, which reveals her feeling trapped in the situation.

Round disk figures were making me do things. Like in one instance I was in a safety pin race with elephants and I was walking so slowly; I couldn't walk fast enough and the elephants would beat me. I re-remember feeling this terror that something terrible would happen if they beat me and each time I would wake up before the end of the race . . . . I couldn't do what I wanted to do . . . I couldn't move fast enough.

Management of Silent Reaction

The definition of silent reaction to accessory to sex is when the child has kept the burden of the secret of the activity within herself. This secret creates considerable tension and victims have several reactions from keeping the secret.

Coconspiracy dyad. Two victims of the same offender agreed that they did not feel guilty about the sexual experience but rather about the fact that they had kept it hidden from the parents. In this situation, when the secret was disclosed, a split occurred in the family and this was equally upsetting to the victim. In another silent reaction the victim said,

It's the lying and the hiding and the not talking about it that is bad. It has to be put into perspective—need to talk about it rather than make it such a hideous thing.

Resistance techniques. There are techniques that children will use to aid in avoiding the sexual activity. They do not betray the secret and they do not disobey the pledge to secrecy, however, but they do play a game. One victim said,

He said I would get another silver dollar if I did it. And I said I did not want to do it right then but that I would do it some other time. And for the next 7 years I played that little game: "Well, I can't do it now, I have to do this for my mother." I was never so diligent for my mother except when we were visiting.

In a situation involving a father and two daughters, one victim described how her sister managed to avoid the father:

My sister said my father was doing the same thing . . . but she wasn't afraid to talk back—be aggressive about it and he left her alone . . . . She would get emotionally sick now that I think back. She would throw up her food when she was upset. She cried a lot and had nightmares—that would be when he was after her and this kept him away from her.

Symptom formation. Symptoms will develop as the person is pressured to keep the secret over time and they are related to the tension inherent in the fear of disclosure. Fears become exaggerated as in the following case:

> I felt anxiety, frustration, and constant fear—a real paranoia that someone would find out. It affected my relationships with my peers. I lived in a shell and escaped by reading. . . . I was always afraid of people and thought something terrible would happen if people found out.

The fear may be exaggerated to the degree that the woman feels that her sexual partners will know she has had such an experience and she may even fear blackmail. One victim said, "I was afraid if I ever told a man or anyone that I might be blackmailed."

Reporting a silent reaction. What triggers the person to reveal to another person the incident is clinically important. It may be a timely question, it may be an association to a conversation, or it may be the concern of the interviewer. One victim said the first person she told was a close friend. It was over the telephone and they were both drunk. Another victim could not tell anyone until the significant parties involved were dead.

One notable feature of when the silence is broken is the characteristic of the unresolved issue phenomenon. The incident has been encapsulated within the psychic structure for so long that when the person finally discloses the secret, the emotional affect can be quite strong as in the following case.

> . . . I am going to get hysterical in a minute and that's really terrible. I always giggle when I get very upset. I'm sorry . . . . You know, he was wearing green work pants with a metal zipper. I never thought of that before either; I never really sat down and discussed it in detail. He unbuttoned his shirt, god . . . and he unbuttoned my blouse . . . all of a sudden I just have this feeling of this hairy chest on my chest . . . like remembering him rubbing my chest . . . with his chest.

When a clinician diagnoses a silent reaction to a sexual trauma situation, the details of the incident should be fully discussed in order to start the process of resolving the incident.

Discussion

In the limited number of research articles on the subject of the psychological components of child victims of sexual offenses, the issues of participation or the child's personality structure are stressed. This is not the intent of this diagnostic category, but rather it is described from the victim's point of view, the dynamics involved between offender and victim regarding the issues of pressure to have sex, secrecy, and disclosure of the secret. It is important to keep in mind that the child does react to being involved in the sexual activity and that the syndrome reaction is one result of the pressure to keep the activity secret.

It may be speculated that there are many children with silent reaction to sexual trauma. The child who responds to the pressure to go along with the sexual activity with an adult may be viewed as showing an adaptive response for survival in the environment. Case finding for this type of sexual child abuse will not be easy.

SEX-STRESS SITUATION

The third type of sexual trauma, the sex-stress situation,[11] is an anxiety reaction that occurs as a result of the circumstances or result of a sexual situation in which both parties consented. The cases are not cases of the male's gaining access without the female's initial consent, nor were they cases in which the victim, for personality or cognitive reasons, was incapable of making a decision of consent. Rather, as each story unfolded, it was clear that the case was one in which the male and female initially agreed to have sexual relations, but then something drastically "went wrong." Usually, what goes wrong is that the male exploits this agreement in several ways. In some cases, what went wrong was that the authorities—police or parents—came upon or found out about the consenting couples; and these authorities themselves either defined the situation as rape or caused the person to say it was rape as a way out of a dilemma of being caught. Also, in some sex-stress cases, the person who referred to the problem as rape in reality wants some service from the hospital and does not know how to ask for it. After all, given the prevailing attitudes, a young teen-ager cannot walk into a hospital and say she and her boyfriend had sex the evening before, she is now scared of becoming pregnant, and she needs medication to prevent a pregnancy. It should be emphasized that very few of these sex-stress victims took the case to court; they did not become "spite cases," that is, cases in which the female sought to "get the guy" on a rape charge simply out of spite.

[11] A. W. Burgess and L. L. Holmstrom, *Rape: Victims of Crisis* (Bowie, Md.: R. J. Brady Company, 1974), pp. 14–19. Reprinted with permission.

It is important for clinicians to understand sex-stress cases for several reasons. First, they greatly influence how the system deals with rape. Staff members tend to become obsessed with trying to determine if a case is a rape case or if it is one of the other types described here. A tremendous amount of energy goes into this type of diagnosing rather than helping the victim with the request for aid. Second, these sex-stress cases deserve counseling in their own right. These females are victims in their own way and have many emotional concerns over what to them has been an upsetting experience. The two main types of sex-stress situations are mutual agreement and contracting for sex.

Mutual Agreement

In the sex-stress situation, both parties have agreed to have sex. Both are willing but then something goes wrong. The male becomes perverted; the female becomes anxious; or the authorities—police or parents—intervene.

Perversion and violence. In the sex-stress victim, what may have happened is that the man became violent or perverted in his approach and frightened the woman. The following example is a case in point. It involves a 47-year-old woman who describes how she met the offender in a lounge. They had considerable conversation leading up to the point where they left the lounge with the purpose of returning to his apartment to have sex there. He had offered to pay her money for the sex, but she said she was not interested in being paid. The woman describes what happened:

> He had given me a good con job and I was looking forward to having sex with him . . . then he took me outside and down an alley and threw me on the ground. I asked him what he was doing—told him he didn't have to do it there . . . he just pulled everything off me . . . I couldn't believe what was happening . . . . He tried natural sex; then he insisted on oral sex . . . . He rammed his fists up me twice and he bit my breasts. Then he stood up and piddled on me and said, "I feel better." . . . He told me not to leave—he hit me and said, "You will do what I say." . . . I started to get dressed and then he was back. He had another guy with him. The guy who raped me asked the other guy if he wanted me and the guy said, "I want no part of it." They both walked away.

Victim's anxiety over sexuality. Occasionally, a female will become so anxious after having sexual relations, especially about getting pregnant, that she may say that a rape occurred. She may report the incident as a rape so that she can be examined and receive medication. For example, a 14-year-old girl came to the hospital accompanied by her girlfriend and stated that she had been raped by two boys the previous evening. She said she came home, did not say anything to her parents, and went to her room. She described the rest of the evening as follows:

> I went to bed but I didn't sleep. I banged on the mirror; I pulled my hair—I just went crazy. I finally lay down and went to sleep for a few hours. I woke at 6 A.M. and went over to my girlfriend's house and woke her up. I got hysterical and told her she had to help me . . . . I figured I could handle this myself if I had my friend to help me. We began reading a book and we began to get scared I might get pregnant. I figured I was midway in my period. I almost blacked out over that. My friend said we could go to a clinic and not have to give our names.

At the hospital, the girl was adamant that her parents or police not be notified. The hospital was unable to treat without parental permission and after 2 hours of talking with all available hospital staff, the girl agreed to have her parents notified. Her mother immediately came to the hospital. The examination indicated no physical trauma, the hymen was still intact, and laboratory tests indicated no sperm present.

On follow-up, the mother revealed that the daughter later had been able to tell her that it was not a rape experience but rather her first sexual contact, and that, plus the possibility of pregnancy, had frightened the girl. Counseling involved talking with the mother and daughter separately in order to help them deal with their feelings and reactions to the situation.

Parental anxiety over sexuality. Parents may become so overwhelmed with worry about their child's sexuality that they, too, may come to the hospital and claim that a rape has occurred in order to have the girl examined. The mother of a 14-year-old girl came to the emergency ward of the hospital and took the nurse aside and said, "My girl was raped 2 days ago. Can you check without telling her you know?"

A talk with the mother revealed some of her concern.

> About 3 weeks ago I noticed a change in her behavior. She was staying out late and a male was calling and identifying himself as "her man." She has been acting strange and suspicious; she doesn't talk

to me. I suspect she is having sex. Why else would she be staying
out so late? . . . I don't feel a 14-year-old girl should be giving her
body to those good-for-nothing boys. She knows I'm strictly against
it. Boys just want one thing.

The gynecologist said that the girl had rights to privacy and that
he would not examine her for virginity reasons. He did say he
would talk with the girl alone to see if she did have some concerns
to talk to him about. It did result in a request from the girl for
birth control pills, and she was referred to the adolescent gynecological clinic at the hospital. In this type of situation, the
mother and daughter were counseled separately, with the goal
being to relieve the anxiety of each one so that a more comfortable and less suspicious relationship could develop between the
two.

Police intervention. There are situations in which police come
upon a parked automobile in which the occupants are engaged in
sexual activity. The girl may have consented. Such a situation
may come to the attention of the hospital staff, however, if the
girl is under age and her anxiety is sufficient to cause her to be
either confused or agitated at the time.

In one situation, a 14-year-old girl went willingly in a car
with two men, one of whom was known to her. The 16-year-old
youth she had been dating was one of the occupants, and the
driver of the car was the 35-year-old uncle. The police happened
onto the car, and the girl said she was forced to have sex with
both of them. The charges were dropped at court the next day
when the mother agreed the girl had gone willingly in the car.
Counseling was important to both the girl and her mother as they
needed to talk over their feelings as well as about future behavior
for the girl.

Parental intervention. There are situations in which the parent perceives some danger to the daughter's reputation and assumes responsibility in the matter. For example, this might happen
if a daughter was missing overnight. The parents become concerned and either notify the police or wait for the daughter to
come home. In such situations, the offenders are often men in
their twenties and thirties and not in the same peer age range as
the girl.

In one situation involving a 13-year-old girl, the foster
mother said,

Joan didn't come home when she was supposed to, so we called the police and reported her as a runaway. Then someone said they had seen her, so her father went looking for her and heard where she was. He told the police but they were unable to find her. Then on Sunday Joan came home to change her clothes—she had new clothes on. She said she was going to a banquet with this boy she met. I called the police and they talked with Joan who took them back to the apartment. They found her clothes and the man was seen running out the back door and across the yard.

In this case, the man was apprehended by the police and charges of statuatory rape were pressed by the parents. The man defaulted at trial level however, and a warrant for his arrest was issued.

Contracting for Sex

A number of prostitutes who contract for sex find out later that their client does not live up to the contract. He becomes perverse, becomes violent, robs her, or does not pay for services obtained. As a result, prostitutes often feel they are in danger and as a result sometimes turn to the police for protection. The police, in turn, bring the woman to the hospital for medical attention. These women often have a number of concerns as the following chapter illustrates.

Management of the Victim of Sex Stress

People who are victimized by a sexually stressful situation are equally deserving of crisis counseling. Although the sexual situation is not a rape situation, where the act is by force and against the victim's will, the person has still been through a situation she has perceived as very upsetting. Or, the situation proves stressful to another person such as a parent. The emotional reaction of the person in distress is that of anxiety and the techniques of aiding a person with anxiety is the most beneficial treatment model. The clinician should fully assess the situation and obtain all the details that will help to put it into perspective for the victim. Then an assessment of the person's coping abilities and social network support is made and an intervention plan according to the results of the data.

SUMMARY

This chapter has discussed three diagnostic categories of sexual trauma. Rape trauma syndrome is an acute stress reaction to a life-threatening situation and includes two distinct phases: the disorganization of the victim's life-style and the reorganization process of putting the life-style back together. The accessory-to-sex syndrome is a situation in which the person is pressured into sexual activity by one of three means: pressure for material goods, pressure by misrepresenting moral standards, and pressure for human contact. The syndrome results from the pressure of keeping the activity secret and the results when the secret is disclosed. Sex-stress situation is an anxiety reaction to a situation which both parties initially consent but then something goes wrong. What goes wrong is the key to the anxiety. Counseling and management aspects of each diagnostic category is discussed.

14

the prostitute

Prostitution has been discussed sociologically, legally, and morally, but seldom from a clinical standpoint. Classroom lectures for health professionals rarely discuss the issue and textbooks fail to include any material that is helpful to the clinician who sees the prostitute in a community setting. In fact, staff personnel who are called upon to interview or examine a prostitute may well wonder what their specific goal is. What type of service is the client seeking, and what should one say to the client?

The lack of specific information that is helpful to health professionals in varying settings coupled with the findings from a project that identified crisis concerns of the prostitute led to the development of this chapter. The study results demonstrated that the presence of prostitutes in the emergency ward of the hospital and at a police station making complaints influences the way people perceive rape victims in general. To some staff who work in a hospital or a police station, the term *rape victim* triggers a suspicious attitude that the victim may not be telling the truth or that she may be a prostitute who wasn't paid.

Sections adapted from A. W. Burgess and L. L. Holmstrom, *Rape: Victims of Crisis* (Bowie, Md.: Robert J. Brady, Company, 1974),and used with permission.

It became clear in talking with police and hospital staff that considerable energy is exerted by people asking themselves, "Is it a real rape, or is she a prostitute?" Second, it became clear that if the time is taken to talk to the prostitute about her problems, one will learn a great deal. The literature on prostitution, like that on rape, has tended to overlook the human predicament of the women involved. Prostitutes have important information to tell and people need to listen and to understand their prospective.

VICTIMIZATION OF THE PROSTITUTE

There are ways in which prostitutes are victimized because of their occupation. This becomes increasingly clear when listening to the prostitute who comes to the emergency ward of a hospital. Prostitutes are exploited in two ways: (1) rape, and (2) sex-stress situations that include nonpayment, perversion, robbery, and violence. Prostitutes are especially vulnerable to exploitation in these ways. Since the services they provide are against the law at present, it is much harder for them to obtain justice when reporting their victimization to the authorities.

Rape

For a man who wants to rape a woman, the prostitute is an easy mark. She is often known by her occupation or by her style of "hooking" or by her hours of work. The prostitute is often on the street in the early hours of the morning when there is minimal protection. Some prostitutes are raped because the man knows who they are. One prostitute in describing her assailant said he had once been a customer of hers when she had been a prostitute and that when she told him she did not hussle anymore, he pulled a gun and said he would "blow my brains out" if I didn't do as he commanded.

Some men know that the prostitute will have an extremely poor chance of going to court and of bringing charges against them due to her own reputation and record with the courts. Many prostitutes resort to "street justice" rather than attempting to bring charges against the man through the criminal justice system. As one prostitute said, "I am going to have my friends get them (the assailants) . . . they will go out looking for all four of them."

A prostitute is sensitive to the idea of many people that because of her occupation she cannot be raped. As one woman said during an emergency room interview following a rape attack,

"Most people say a prostitute can't be raped, but I believe in my heart I was. I feel so dirty by the whole experience . . . not like I do when I do it for money."

There are two ways that the prostitute may be approached by the man. The first is where the man attempts to make direct contract for sex and the prostitute turns him down. One victim recounts her experience as follows.

> I had met the man before and knew him from the group at the bar. One afternoon I was with some of my girlfriends . . . he came over and started talking . . . . He loud mouthed me . . . he wanted to give me money to use my body. The waitress saw he was annoying me and came over and told him to get away . . . . Later I went outside and started to go home . . . . Next thing I knew I was grabbed by my neck and pushed into an alley. I screamed and he put his hand over my mouth. Then he pushed me into a window and down into a room that was covered with broken glass and bottles. I kept screaming . . . he ripped my clothes off. I took glass to hit him and then got scared and dropped it. He beat my head and told me to shut up . . . . I heard guys outside yelling for him to hurry up and he told me they were waiting their turn.

In this case, police officers arrived on the scene after receiving a call that a woman was screaming in the area. The police officer testified at the court hearing that he heard a woman yelling, "Help me. Someone please help me." When the officer flashed his light into the window, he saw the assailant and ordered him out. After advising the man of his rights, the man said, "Hey, that's what makes the world go round. I gave her $12." Later at the police station when he was being booked he said, "You have me wrong. I gave her $20." No money of either quantity was found on the woman. The case did proceed through superior court and resulted in a hung jury but the woman refused to go through the court process again. By this time the defense lawyer had learned of her prostitution history and had been prepared to base his case on this knowledge for the second trial.

A second way in which a prostitute may be approached is by being well-known in her occupation. The following case illustrates this type.

> Nora, a 22-year-old attractive woman wearing a frosted wig and brown hot pants, tan jersey, and a blue multicolor design blazer, was brought to the emergency service by the police at 5 A.M. She was barefoot; the men had taken her black suede platform sandal shoes. She cried when describing certain parts of the experience but was composed and in control of her reactions for most of the interview.

Nora said she was walking along the street after leaving a local bar, when a small car pulled up and a little man jumped out, grabbed her by the arm, and pulled her into the car. He put his arm around her neck and said, "We want to fuck you." The man driving the car spoke in a foreign language to the other man. When they arrived at the apartment building, the man put his hand over Nora's mouth and pushed her up to a third-floor apartment. In the apartment, the men told her to take her clothes off. She said no, and one man started to pull at her clothes and jacket, and the other man slapped her in the face and punched her in the chest. The men seemed to fight with each other over who was to be first. The big man pushed the little one, which angered him to the point that he put on all his clothes which he had already taken off; he took Nora's shoes and money—$6—that she had in her purse. He threatened to take everything as he left and said, "How'd you like to go home without your clothes and hair?"

The big man pushed Nora on the bed and asked how much money she made a night and what she charged. Then he asked her to blow him and threatened to cut her up in little pieces and leave her in the cellar if she did not do as he said. She was quite frightened by this. The man said he wanted sex. Nora said she had her period and that she had a tampon in place. This did not matter to him and the man continued to penetrate her. Nora told him he was hurting her, which made no difference.

The little man then came back to the apartment and the two men began shouting at each other. The little man took a candle and beat Nora with it—said he did that because a candle would leave no marks (and it did not).

Nora finally managed to get away from the men and went to a security guard at a local restaurant; he called the police who in turn brought her to the hospital. The police, who knew her, said the facts indicated that she had been raped. The two men were arrested and the case was assigned to a hearing. Typical of the other prostitutes who were able to identify the assailant who raped, robbed, or assaulted them, however, this woman never appeared in court. The decision not to appear seemed to occur with the prostitutes who were known to the police and who had arrests for prostitution. It is speculated that they feel their backgrounds would be held against them. This is one reason why, in the majority of these cases, the woman does not appear for district-level hearings and the case is usually dismissed.

Sex-Stress Situations

Prostitution is basically a business transaction involving an agreement between the provider and the buyer. The prostitute offers services for a price and the customer who obtains the services is expected to pay for them. Customers may, however, violate the verbal contract by nonpayment, perversion, violence, or robbery. Many of the prostitutes seen in the emergency ward had been victims of such sexually stressful situations during the course of the night's work. It should be noted, however, that the chief complaint of these victims, as listed in the hospital record, is *rape.* Societal attitudes and the law are such that one does not simply walk into the hospital and say, "I work the streets and something really upsetting happened to me tonight." Instead, the patient must make the request for help in an indirect way. Thus, for official bureaucratic purposes the chief complaint is listed as *rape.*

Nonpayment. Prostitutes are aware of the possibility that they might not be paid. Some will say, for example, that as a precaution they always try to obtain the money before providing the sex. Nevertheless, nonpayment is still a common form of exploitation. It seems to occur in the following ways.

First, as in the opening example, the man persuades the woman to have sex and then he refuses to pay. One prostitute said she had been persuaded to provide sex first because the man had said, "The last time I paid first, the girl took the money and left and I got nothing." Or, if it is a group of men and several prostitutes, one man may say the other man is paying, and because of the circumstances of the situation the woman is never paid.

Second, the contract is made and then violence is used instead of money. There may be two men, one of whom holds the woman while the other forces her to have sex and then the roles are reversed. The woman is then pushed out of the car and no money is paid. Or, after the contract is made there is a weapon used rather than payment.

Perversion. Prostitutes typically have a certain range of sexual services that they sell, but these do not necessarily include the full gamut of what certain men desire. Thus, the prostitute may find out only when it is too late that the customer really has much more in mind than she does.

Robbery. Prostitutes are easy prey for robbery. They are known by their occupation and may keep their money with them until the end of the night's work. Thus, victims may complain of being robbed.

Violence. Prostitutes become equally concerned when the sexual behavior of the client turns to violence. They say very explicitly that they fear for their lives when this occurs. As one woman said, "I'll go to court on this one. I hope they hang him. This time the guy beat me up and he's a sadist. Suppose he got a virgin sometime—it could ruin her mentally." The woman went on to describe parts of the assault:

> He said he would kill me if I didn't do as he said. He called me names such as whore, cunt, slut. Then he would ask me if I was scared while he waved the gun in my face. Then he asked me if I would like it if he killed himself in front of me—would it be an experience for me?

REACTIONS TO VICTIMIZATION

A Range of Emotions

Prostitutes respond to rape, nonpayment, violence, and other types of victimization with a variety of feelings. Some link their reaction specifically to their feelings of being exploited as a woman. One prostitute said, "The man said I didn't have to put the police onto him. But he doesn't know how I felt as a woman. I had to get some revenge. I had to do something. He forced me to have sex."

Another prostitute said, "I feel I was used, treated like a joke, treated like an animal. It was inhuman." Such statements often come from women who have been forced to indulge in what they regard as perverse sexual acts or who have been degraded in very specific terms or sent into the street without any clothes.

It is not unusual to find the prostitute very angry and wishing for some revenge. One woman intended to find her assailants and stated

> I am going to stand around (street walking) till I see them again. Then I am going to tell the police. I will stand around till I see them. I have already told the police the first half of the license plate, and I just need to find the rest of the number or the guys.

Revenge can take another route with a different type of weapon. One prostitute who was concerned that she might have a venereal disease said, "Maybe they'll catch it. I hope they suffer. They won't notice they have it (until it is too late). They were so out on dope."

Ambivalence about Being "In the Life"

In contrast to the prostitutes quoted above, whose concern was with the particular victimization that had just occurred, some of the prostitutes also voiced concern about their life-styles. The prostitutes who did this tended to be ambivalent about being "in the life" and seemed to be trying to decide if prostitution was what they really wanted to do. Their comments focused not only on the exploitation aspect but also on their own reactions to being a prostitute and the reactions of other people to their occupation. They were reacting to a more diffuse kind of victimization—that which results from living in a society where some people are only too willing to reward them for their services and others berate them for these same services. Ambivalence was also shown in another case in which a woman contracted for sex but then at the last moment could not go through with the act. This woman stated

> I've just arrived in Boston and I was looking for an apartment—a cheap one. Two men were on the street. I asked them if they knew of any apartments and we talked, and then after awhile they offered me a ride back to where I was staying. While in the car they propositioned me and said each would pay me $15. We went to their apartment, but I just couldn't go through with it. I told them and tried to get away. The older guy didn't care, but the younger man forced me to have sex. I couldn't get away from him.

In the following case, the woman volunteered the information about her work and her reactions to it:

> I had thought of going to the street for a profession. Thought about it and ended up doing it . . . . Did it today, but it was just one of those days. But I go for my checkups; clean myself out; don't take any chances. I am living with a girlfriend. My mother said if I went into that, she might as well forget that she had a daughter. She said if she died, not to come to the funeral. I wanted my daughter to live with me, but my mother kept her—said she would understand things.

This woman's reaction was: "I will have to be more cautious. I am edgy now; nerves are bad. Get these awful sinus headaches." She also reported that she had been seeing a psychiatrist. She had taken an overdose of pills and prior to hospital discharge saw the psychiatrist. When asked if she had someone to talk to about the sex-stress incident, the woman replied, "Maybe I should talk about it. Gives me a headache to keep it inside. I try to keep on the bright side and not make things seem so bad." Not only did the woman express her ambivalence about her life-style but she was also aware of the tension her life-style created in her life. This woman talked spontaneously to the victim counselor and clearly indicated a request to ventilate.

MANAGEMENT

It appears that the prostitute may experience a crisis situation in her work not only when raped but when she is victimized by a sexually stressful situation. Some of the specific therapeutic skills that are useful in aiding the prostitute during the crisis are as follows.

1. *Listen for the crisis request.* Although the prostitute may be quickly labeled by the hospital staff or police, this label tells nothing of her request for aid. The clinician will learn more of the reason she has come for aid if the woman is dealt with in a straight respectful manner. It is too easy to jump to conclusions and to judge the woman prior to listening and reviewing her account of the incident carefully as she has perceived it.

Following the same interview guide used with victims is the best method as this approach conveys to the woman that she is important, that her request for aid is being respected, and that she is being listened to carefully. Such an approach may elicit valuable information that reveals her occupation. With such information, the clinician is in a better position to talk about the problems of this type of work and to encourage the prostitute to talk about them.

2. *Encouraging dialogue.* Generally, the woman must tell the clinician that she does work the streets for the counseling to be most meaningful. It is interesting to note how many prostitutes will talk of their life-style when given the time and the interest by the counselor. Although they may not want follow-up, their wish to talk at the hospital indicates a request to ventilate. If staff are available to see such women at the hospital, there might be more understanding of the problems of their occupation.

3. *Bearing painful feelings.* Prostitutes belong to a specific subcultural group and usually obtain emotional support from

the group. They do suffer, however, from the attitudes of society and judgmental opinions of professional people who are called upon to treat them. It may be assumed that they have feelings about their rejection from society and especially feelings about admitting their work to professionals.

The prostitutes were sufficiently upset when seen at the hospital; some cried while waiting for the interview or during their discussion of the evening's events. The degrading experience they have endured as a result of the sexually stressful situation evokes considerable feelings in many of the women. Therefore, one therapeutic task is to help bear the feelings with them. Painful feelings for prostitutes are often humiliation, degrading accusations, and society's reaction to them.

4. *Implementing the medical model.* The prostitute is quite vulnerable to medical problems such as venereal disease. Many women have health checks regularly but many do not. Gynecological examination may reveal venereal disease, pelvic inflammatory disease, and vaginal infections. It is good clinical practice for all clinicians to encourage the woman to keep herself in close medical supervision, and recommending the hospital clinic or other resources is very important during the initial interview.

SUMMARY

It has been stated that prostitution is a big business in the United States, yet little is known about the prostitute herself and the problems she encounters in her occupation. Often prostitutes come to the accident floor of the hospital stating that they have been raped. In talking with these women about their problems, it was concluded that some were the victims of rape and others were victims of their clients through nonpayment, perversion, robbery, and violence. In many cases, the prostitute herself sought police and medical intervention. It was found also that a number of the prostitutes were upset by their recent experience—whether it be rape or sex stress—and did wish to talk to someone about their feelings. By "playing it straight" and listening for their request, counselors can provide services to a group, namely prostitutes, that in general has not been reached before.

index